12 lessons of wellness & weightloss

for kids and teens

Workbook

12 lessons for today's kids and teens who want to grow into a healthy weight. Breaking down the huge topic of weight loss into 12 lessons brings you many opportunities to approach healthy habits from a variety of angles. You will also have participants returning for more education, learning how to stay on track, and even having a little fun in lighthearted competitions. You can use the 12 Lessons over a month, a few months or even a year.

By Food and Health Communications, Inc. with food log makeovers by Victoria Shanta Retelny, RD.

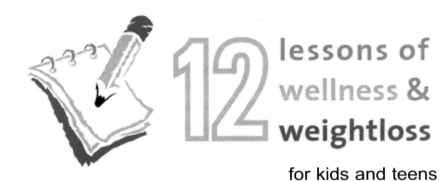

12 lessons of wellness & weightloss

for kids and teens

For more cooking information, visit us online:
www.foodandhealth.com

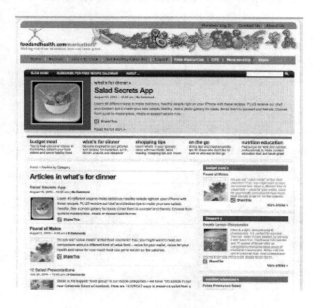

Download our new Salad Secrets App for the iPhone and find over 50 of our best salad recipes (with photos!). You can even email them to clients right from your phone.

12 Lessons of Wellness and Weight Loss for Teens

This 12 lesson plan for weight loss breaks goals into 12 easy, relevant lessons based on the Dietary Guidelines for Americans and MyPlate.

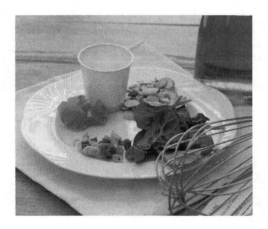

Food and Health Communications, Inc.
Louisville, Colorado
www.foodandhealth.com

Food and Health Communications

P.O. Box 271108

Louisville, CO 80027

www.foodandhealth.com

Copyright 2013 Food and Health Communications

Printed in the United States

This book is printed in ebook, epub, workbook and CD-ROM for-

mats. For special licensing, contact Food and Health

Communications at 800-462-2352 or through

their website at foodandhealth.com

ISBN-13: 978-1490393810

ISBN-10: 1490393811

Table of Contents

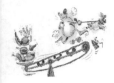

Obesity is on the Rise

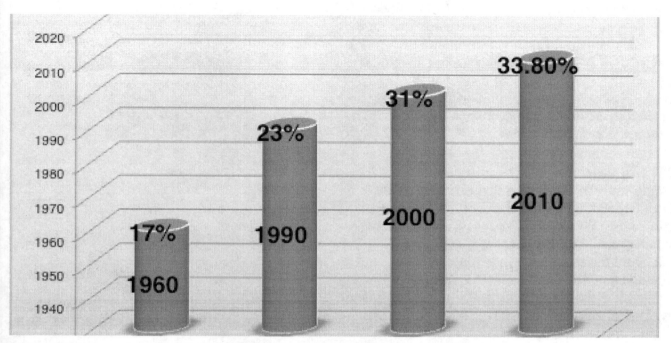

Calorie Consumption is Increasing

Americans now eat 523 more calories per day than they did in 1970. Additionally lifestyles in the U.S, have become less physically active and provide little opportunity to burn off those excess calories. The result? Skyrocketing obesity rates. Just look at the graph above!

Obesity-Related Health Problems

When you weigh much more than you should, you put extra strain on your heart, lungs, muscles, bones, etc. In fact, obesity is currently considered the second leading cause of preventable death in the United States. A few of the health risks associated with obesity are listed below...

- Diabetes
- Gallbladder
- Heart Disease
- Osteoarthritis
- Sleep apnea

Obesity is Officially on the Map

The chart below illustrates the percentage of obese adults in each state.

Increasing obesity rates have crawled across the map over the years. In 1985, there wasn't a single state that had obese people as more than a quarter of its population. In 2010 there were more than 30 states at least that percentage! What does your home state look like? What percentage of the population is obese?

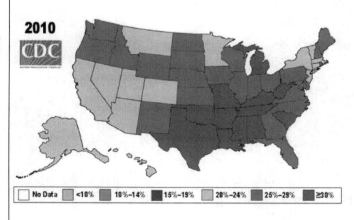

7

Consume Fewer Calories

There are lots of ways to consume fewer calories. Why not try to eat smaller, more frequent meals and use smaller dishes, bowls, and cups? If you crave a second helping, go back for salads or vegetables. You can also arrange your plate into the proportions recommended by MyPlate, and heed their advice about avoiding oversized portions

Eat Smaller, More Frequent Meals

One study demonstrated that eating smaller, more frequent meals aided weight control better than eating one or two large meals during the day. Smaller meals that are eaten frequently also help you avoid the starve-and-stuff routine that is so common among dieters.

Produce For Everyone!

Eat more fruits and vegetables. After all, they're generally low-calorie and high-fiber foods. You can also use fruits and veggies to displace higher-calorie foods by eating a salad before lunch and dinner. You can sub fruits and veggies for high calorie processed foods like cookies and crackers too.

Choose Low Calorie Whole Grains

Choose cooked whole grains instead of refined grains. Did you know that cooked grains are lowest in calorie density? Just look at the calorie density of these sample foods...

Cooked oatmeal	0.6
Cooked rice	.9
Whole-wheat bread	2.6
Crackers	4.3

Consume Fewer Dairy Calories

Choose low-fat or skim dairy products and beware of items with a lot of added sugar. Yogurt, frozen yogurt, skim milk, and lowfat cheese are all good choices.

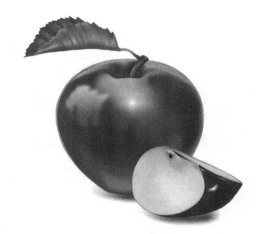

Consume Fewer Protein Calories

Eat small portions of a variety of beans, meat, fish, and poultry. Choose lean items and keep them low in fat. That means no frying or drenching in butter. Instead, try broiling, grilling, or baking them.

More Tips, Fewer Calories

- Eat only when you're actually hungry.
- Limit the number of sweets you eat.
- Limit the number of fatty foods you eat.
- Read food labels.

Be Aware of What You're Eating

Try writing down what you eat in a day. This will help you be aware of how many calories you consume. 3,500 excess calories consumed adds up to 1 pound of body fat gained. An extra 50 calories a day, every single day, will result in a five-pound weight gain by the end of the year.

Real awareness of what and when you eat will help you make better choices. Often, people have one or two trouble foods that trigger them to overindulge. Maybe yours is a bag of potato chips or a large cookie, or just bad choices when you eat out. See if you can find a lower-calorie alternative for these foods. A registered dietitian can be a fantastic resource for battling trigger foods. Visit *eatright.org* for more information.

Exercise and Move More

There are lots of ways to lose weight. Try eating 300 fewer calories than you would need in order to maintain your current weight. Increase the amount of physical activity you do each day until you are burning off an additional 200 calories.

Taking these steps should result in a weight loss of one pound per week. Gradual weight loss promotes long-term loss of body fat, not just the water weight that is quickly regained. It should also involve portion control and proper diet, but here we're going to focus on the other part of the equation: exercise. Learn how to be active. That way you will burn more calories AND become physically fit.

People are Less Active

In this day and age, lifestyles are less active, because...

- More jobs are accomplished via computer.
- Labor-saving devices are more prevalent.
  - Garage door openers
  - Dishwashers
  - Washing machines, dryers
  - Microwaves
  - Power tools
  - Maid and lawn services
  - Televisions and computers

Compare the way that we live our lives to the lifestyles of our great-grandparents. For example, many people now do the majority of their work behind a computer. How did previous generations earn a salary? Also, try to imagine how many calories must have been burned carrying water or chopping wood. What devices have saved us from doing those same chores? Finally, consider transportation. How do our methods of getting from one place to another differ from those used in years past?

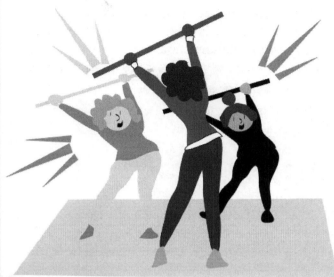

Did You Know?

- You burn double the number of calories when you move around instead of sitting still.
- Cleaning the house burns 152 calories per hour, while sitting burns just 76 calories per hour.
- Starting an exercise routine too quickly can lead to injury or burnout. Start slow and work your way up to tougher activities.

Burn Those Calories!

- Exercise for an hour, most days of the week.
- Lift weights or do some other kind of resistance training a few times per week.

The Dietary Guidelines for Americans insist that, in order to lose weight and keep it off, people need to exercise for 60-90 minutes per day on most days of the week. You can reach this exercise goal in a single, long, daily workout, or in small bursts throughout the day.

Sample 60 Minute Workout

- Cleaning the house – 10 minutes
- Walking briskly at lunch – 10 minutes
- Exercising with a home video – 40 minutes

Total: 60 minutes

More Ways to Exercise

Ways to Move More Often
- Take the stairs rather than the elevator whenever you have the choice.
- Walk to nearby places you want to visit – the mall, a friend's house, etc.
- Volunteer or enroll in after school activitites, especially sporting events.

Take a Pedometer for a Spin
- 6,000 steps = Average daily steps
- 8,000 steps = 1 extra mile = 100 calories
- 10,000 steps = 2 extra miles = 200 calories
- 12,000 steps = 3 extra miles = 300 calories

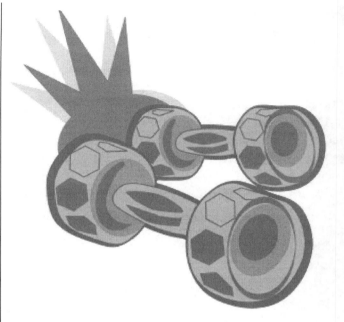

Measure Your Steps
The average person takes about 6,000 steps each day. 2,000 steps is about the same as traveling one mile, and walking one mile burns 100 calories. By increasing steps per day to 8,000, a person can burn an extra 100 calories. Taking 10,000 steps/day increases calories burned to 200 calories each day (Source: Raussin et al, JCI 1986).

Activity Levels Affect Weight Gain
According to Dr. James Hill of the University of Colorado's Health and Science Center, the vast differences between the weights of different people are significantly affected by how active they are in their daily lives.

Hill's study was intense and very controlled. His subjects lived in room calorimeters, which revealed the number of calories that they actually burned in a day. After calorie intake was accurately measured, Hill discovered the largest difference between the number of calories burned was not in the resting metabolic rates of his subjects, but in the amount of work that they performed.

The difference between subjects ranged from 200 to 1,000 calories a day. If there is this much difference between individuals living in a con-fined environment, think about the differences between individuals going about their daily lives in the real world.

Eric Ravussin obtained similar results in his experiment, which also featured a room calorimeter. The number of calories that his subjects burned varied by 100-800 calories... per day!

Start Slow and be Consistent
If you haven't been active, start slowly and work your way up to a healthy amount of daily exercise. Prioritize exercise.

> " ... the most important factor of all is the determination of the American people to overcome the converging forces of poor diets and lack of exercise."
>
> — Joseph Jen, Undersecretary for Research, Education, and Economics, U.S. Department of Agriculture

Case Study: No Time to Plan

Meet NoTime

NoTime is a man in his early 20s

Height	6'1"
Weight	270
BMI	36
BMI category	Obesity II
Waist Circumference	42"

Notes

NoTime presented to a registered dietitian (RD) a bit reluctantly. He was worried about having to making changes and did not like strict rules. He thrived on chaos and was constantly running from one thing to the next. Needless to say, he did not plan his meals or snacks. His constant tiredness was finally getting to him, and he claimed to have no time for physical activity.

Upon nutrition assessment, the RD noted that NoTime grabbed whatever was available when he was hungry. He typically ate "something" at meal times – even if it didn't constitute a meal. For example, he thought nothing of grabbing a donut or an Egg Mcmuffin for breakfast. Sometimes he chose salads – but they were often high calorie creations like taco salads. He had been physically active in high school sports, but once he went away to college, his physical activity waned and his eating patterns became worse.

Food Log Revelations

What did NoTime's food log reveal? Basically, there was no rhyme or reason to NoTime's eating habits. He didn't include food quantities in his log and ate at a variety of odd times. He would skip dinner, but then eat something late at night, which ostensibly ruined his appetite for breakfast the next morning. His lack of planning also cost a lot of money, since he bought prepared foods and did very little grocery shopping.

Nutrition Assessment:

Upon looking at the composition of NoTime's diet, his lack of planning appeared to be taking a serious toll on his life. He was not paying the slightest bit of attention to calorie or fat content. His erratic mealtimes did not help his health at all. He needed to start planning more meals and learn what to look for at the grocery store. He also needed education on what to eat at fast food restaurants. Plus, he needed some kind of motivation to begin a regular exercise program.

A Typical Day in the Life of NoTime

Breakfast   **9 AM**   460 calories
Bagel w/ cream cheese + coffee w/ cream

Lunch   **1:00 PM**   830 calories
1 Taco Salad with shell from Taco Bell + 1 diet coke

Snack   **2:00 PM**   280 calories
1 Snickers (from vending machine)

Dinner   **10:00 PM**   760 calories
Personal Pizza Hut "Sausage Lover's" pizza + 2 lite beers

Total Calories In = 2,550! (96 grams fat)

Activities: No regular activity
Total exercise calories out = 0

Calories In – Calories Out = 2,550
Total Daily Calories = 2,550

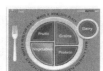

Case Study: No Time to Plan (Part 2)

Nutrition Recommendations:

1. Plan three meals per day and one or two snacks. By eating regular meals, the metabolism stays active and engaged. NoTime should plan to eat every 3 to 4 hours, though meals do not have to be elaborate or expensive. The RD provided a list of healthy grocery store basics, as well as a snack guide and calorie book. These resources made it easy for NoTime to look up food items and quickly assess calorie and fat content. Snacks should be between 100 to 150 calories, and fat should be less than 30% of the total calories consumed.

2. Drink more fluids. The RD advised NoTime to drink water with every meal and snack. Plus, she recommended carrying a water bottle at all times (especially in class). His water consumption goal became 64 oz of water (or decaf/sugar-free beverages) every day.

3. Keep daily food logs to monitor ALL calories. This requires some work on his part because he isn't a planner. The most important thing he can do is write his food intake down. 1) It's right in front of him and 2) It reflects his schedule. The

RD would then review his food logs with him at every visit.

4. Increase physical activity. The RD encouraged NoTime to join a gym on campus or start using the track. He was originally instructed to aim for 30 minutes of physical activity every day. In addition, the RD encouraged NoTime to start weight training in order to build muscle mass.

Outcome:

Over the course of one year, NoTime lost almost 20% of his body weight (and 2" in his waist), which was quite a significant drop. He is still losing weight daily. He started planning meals by going grocery shopping once a week and stocking up on fresh produce, lean protein, and whole grains. His calorie intake dropped to fairly low levels, but the RD recommended nothing under 1200 calories. With his physical activity increasing, NoTime needed to fuel up with sufficient calories. He kept a daily food log on his palm pilot, which made it constantly accessible. Most importantly, NoTime had renewed energy and was sleeping better at night.

A New Day for NoTime

Breakfast	**9:00 AM**	318 calories
1 bagel, 2 Tbs lite cream cheese, 1 slice Canadian bacon, 1 coffee with ½ c. skim milk, 8 oz water		
Snack	**11 AM**	200 calories
1 Chocolate Balance Bar, 8 oz. water		
Lunch	**12:30 PM**	410 calories
Subway turkey breast sandwich (no mayo), small baked chips, 1 diet cola, 8 oz water		
Snack	**3:00 PM**	150 calories
1 McDonald's ice cream cone		
Dinner	**7:00 PM**	460 calories
Healthy Choice Supreme Pizza, side salad w/ lite dressing, 8 oz water		
Snack	**9:30 PM**	165 calories
1 small apple + 1 tablespoon peanut butter, 8 oz water		**Total Calories In = 1,703**
Activity	Bike riding 1 hour (to and from work)	**Total Calories Out = 420**

Food Log

_____ Number of calories per day to maintain my weight.

Determine the number of calories that you need for your current height and weight. To lose a pound a week, you'll need a deficit of 500 calories per day.

Date: _____

Time: **Type and Quantity of Food:**   **Calories Consumed:**

_____

_____

_____

_____

_____

_____

_____

_____

_____

_____

_____

_____

_____

_____   **Total Calories Consumed:** _____

Exercise or strenuous activity (and how long it took):
Calories burned:

_____

_____

_____

_____

_____   **Total Calories Burned:** _____

_____ **Total consumed - total burned = total calories for the day:** _____

Record the day of the week, then enter what you eat during the day in the order in which you ate/drank it. Include all beverages, "tastes," and snacks. To determine calories consumed or burned, use the calculator at _www.caloriecontrol.org_ or go to _www.nutrition.gov_ for information about the calorie content of various foods.

GO! Foods

GO! Foods Are The Best Choices

- Skim milk
- Beans
- Oatmeal
- Stir-fry
- Pasta

- Salad
- Fruit
- Baked potatoes
- Soup

GO!
Best choices for weight control

Vegetables, fruits
Potatoes (low in fat)
Nonfat dairy
Cooked whole grains
Lean protein, legumes

What do GO! foods have in common?

- High in water
- High in fiber
- Low in calorie density
- Low in fat
- No added sugar

GO! foods generally have high water content. This means that cooked whole grains like oatmeal, brown rice, barley, and whole grain pasta are better choices than lower-moisture items like bread and crackers. It's not that bread and crackers are bad for you, they just shouldn't make up the bulk of your diet.

Fruits and vegetables are the best choices for good health and weight loss. They are high in water content and fiber, while low in calorie density and fat. Remember, MyPlate insists that half your plate should be filled with fruits and veggies at each meal. GO! Foods include: fruits, vegetables, nonfat dairy, cooked whole grains, lean protein, and legumes.

What is calorie density?

Calorie density is the concentration of calories in a given weight of food. You can compare foods by grams, ounces, pounds or kilos.

Item	Calories per pound
lettuce	77
apple	224
potato, baked	320
cheese	**1824**
potato chips	**2432**
olive oil	**4000**

See how the **more refined and higher-fat foods are higher in calorie density** than the unprocessed ones?

GO! foods are right in line with the recommendations from the Dietary Guidelines for Americans and MyPlate. They are healthy and often filled with vitamins, minerals, and nutrients. Be sure to eat a wide variety every day... just keep an eye on their size. Stick to MyPlate's advice and avoid oversized portions.

CAUTION! Foods

CAUTION!

High in fat, low in fiber

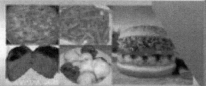

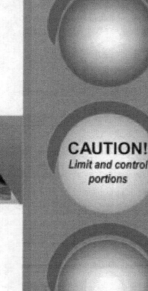

CAUTION!
Limit and control portions

Fatty meats
Fast food
Ice cream, fruit pie

- Pie
- French fries
- Burgers

- Ice cream
- Pizza
- Fatty meats

Caution foods are high in calorie density because they contain a fair amount of fat and only a little moisture. They usually don't have much fiber either. However, these are probably the foods that most Americans eat on a regular basis every day. They are plentiful, fast and easy to grab. They look yummy and taste great. All this makes them dangerous for dieters. However, with a little caution, you can enjoy them in small amounts... as long as you are eating a base of the right stuff. Exercise is also the key to balancing this equation.

Most people would not think of cheesecake as diet food, but they do not realize that pizza, burgers, and fries are in the same calorie-density range as cheesecake.

Being aware of the calorie density of foods makes it easier to make the right choices at home or in a restaurant. You just have to work on using portion control with CAUTION! foods.

It is not that you can never eat a burger and fries. You just need to order small portions. For example, take a look at the calorie content of these three fast food options...

Hamburger	260
Double cheeseburger	730
Big Mac	560

Which is the healthist option? While you shouldn't choose a burger every day, it is possible to indulge without sending the calorie count off the charts.

Some of the foods on the CAUTION! list are good for you and should be consumed in small portions. We're talking about salmon and other fatty fish here, along with things like dried fruit. Eat them in moderation as part of a balanced diet and you'll be all set.

STOP! Foods

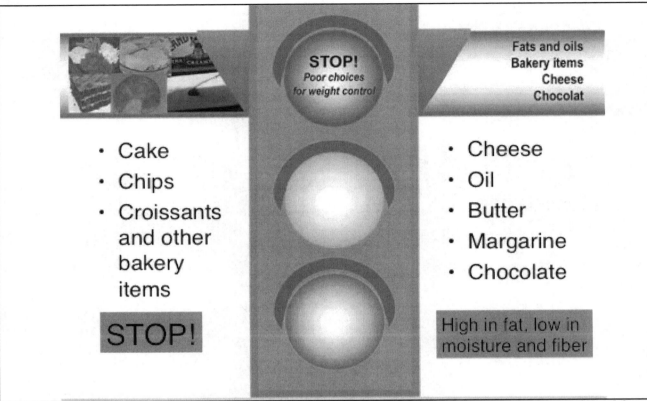

The STOP! foods should be avoided when you are trying to lose weight. They are calorie dense and very high in fat. When you're eating these foods, it is easy to eat too many calories, yet not feel full. You could also stuff yourself and then feel awful. We recommend that you eat STOP! foods very rarely.

Most people are surprised to see that fat-free potato chips, fat-free cakes, and fat-free pretzels rate so high on the calorie-density scale. Fat-free cakes and other baked goods are calorie dense and nutrient poor. They should be avoided if you want to control your weight.

Bread sticks, dry cereals, and crackers are here too. This is because most are made with white flour and do not contain any moisture, which makes them more calorie dense than their moisture rich counterparts.

Oils rate the highest on the calorie density scale (4,000 calories per pound!). There is no water in any of these oils, but there is quite a lot of fat. What does this mean for you? Use it rarely! Measuring spoons and oil spray bottles can help you stay on track.

Nuts and seeds are very nutritious, but still extremely high in fat and calories. While they're a healthier choice than many other STOP! foods, they should be eaten in moderation. The same applies to whole grain bakery items like bread. Use portion control and make these a part of a diet that contains mostly GO! foods.

White flour and white sugar are about the same calorie density. This is why baked goods like cookies are so high in calorie density. They contain white flour, white sugar, and fat. Even when you get rid of the fat, cookies are not much lower in calories because the fat is replaced with more white flour and sugar, along with other ingredients. This is why fat-free foods are not that different (calorie-wise) than their regular counterparts!

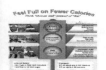

Quick Quiz: What Makes You Full?

Quick Quiz – Do You Know?

- How many oranges would you have to eat to equal the calories in one Snicker's Bar?
- **Snickers Bar = 280 calories**
- **Orange = 61 calories**
- **(Answer: Roughly 4.5 oranges!!)**

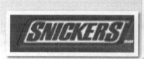

How many oranges would you have to eat in order to equal the calories in one Snickers bar?

Calorie content hints:

Snickers Bar = 280 calories

Orange = 61 calories

Answer: You would have to eat 4.5 oranges!

Do you really think you could eat 4.5 oranges in one sitting? Which do you think would make you feel more full—the 280 calories in the Snickers bar or the 280 calories in the 4.5 oranges?

This is an example of why foods that are high in fiber and low in calorie density are a better choice for weight management. It is hard to consume too many calories when you are choosing items like oranges in place of things like Snickers bars.

Eat oranges, not candy.

Meet the Satiety Index

The satiety index was created by researchers who watched what people ate and recorded how those foods affected how full people felt, along with how much they ate at later meals.

This index shows that high-fat, high-sugar, processed foods that are calorie dense (such as cake, donuts, and candy) are not as filling as foods that are higher in fiber and moisture (such as whole-wheat pasta, potatoes, lentils, baked beans, fruits, and vegetables).

In other words, in order to feel full, you would need to eat more calories from Snickers bars to than you would if you ate things like oranges. Stick to foods that are lower in fat and sugar, yet higher in fiber, and save those candy bars for a special, rare treat.

For more information about calorie density and nutrient density, go to *www.health.gov* and click on the Dietary Guidelines tab.

Go: Best Choices

Category	Products	Calories per pound
Vegetables	all	65-195
Fruits	all except avocado	135-425
Nonfat dairy	skim milk, nonfat yogurt	180-400
Egg whites	whites, egg substitute	226
Nonfat cheese	fat-free cheese	500
High-fiber carbs	potato, peas, beans, yams, corn	300-600
Cooked grains	pasta, rice, barley, cooked cereals	300-600
Lean protein	lean poultry, lean fish, shellfish	450-650

Caution: Use Portion Control!

Category	Products	Calories per pound
Protein	lean beef, salmon, tuna, swordfish	900-1000
Bread	bread, bagels, rolls	1000-1500
Fruit	dried fruit, jams	1000-1500
Fast food	french fries, pizza, burgers	1000-1500
Desserts	cheesecake, apple pie, ice cream	1000-1500
Fatty meats	fatty lunch meats, hot dogs	1000-1500

Stop: Go Very Easy on These

Category	Products	Calories per pound
Fat-free treats	fat-free potato chips, fat-free cakes	1500-2000
Refined carbs	muffins, cookies, fat-free pretzels	1500-2000
Refined carbs	bread sticks, dry cereals, crackers	1500-2000
Cheese	cheddar cheese, Swiss, Brie, etc.	1500-2000
Egg yolks	egg yolks	1500-2000
Regular treats	refined potato chips, cookies, candy carbohydrates brownies, fudge, salad dressing, regular crackers	1500-2500
High-fat products	chocolate candy, nuts &seeds, coconut, peanut butter	2500-3000
High-fat products	bacon, margarine, butter, mayo	3000-3500
Fats and oils	olive oil, lard, vegetable oil, shortening	4000

Label Reading Tip

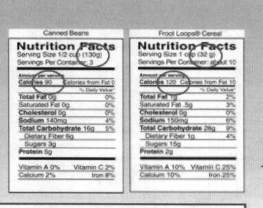

Label Reading Tip

If there are fewer calories than grams per serving, then the food has a low calorie density.

Which food is lower in calorie density?

Did you know that you can determine calorie density simply by looking at a Nutrition Facts label? It's true! If there are fewer calories than grams per serving, that food has a low calorie density. Take a look at these two examples. Which is lower in calorie density?

Canned beans	130 g	90 calories
Sweetened cereal	32 g	122 calories

The beans have a lower calorie density. See how the number of grams per serving is greater than the number of calories per serving?

Calorie density alone does not make a food more delicious. After all, a pound of fresh strawberries is much more palatable than a pound of shortening. The strawberries are just 137 calories per pound, while the shortening is 4,040 calories per pound. Who would want to eat straight shortening anyway?

By increasing your intake of high-fiber fruits and vegetables, you can have a satisfying diet and still lose weight.

Here are some examples of great-tasting GO! foods that are low in calorie density, but high in flavor...

- Soups, stews, chili
- Pasta dishes
- Rice dishes
- Stir-fry dishes
- Baked potatoes
- Fruits
- Steamed vegetables
- Salads with lowfat dressings

Remember to stick to lowfat options and preparations to keep foods healthy. Too much fat content kicks foods right out of the GO! category.

This doesn't mean you have to give up all of the foods you love. You just need to consume them in the right portions. Eat more GO! foods and fewer CAUTION! and STOP! foods.

GO! Foods Puzzle

GO! foods are your best bet for better health and for weight control. They are high in moisture and fiber so they make you feel fuller on fewer calories. GO! foods include fruits, vegetables, nonfat dairy, cooked whole grains, and lean protein and legumes.

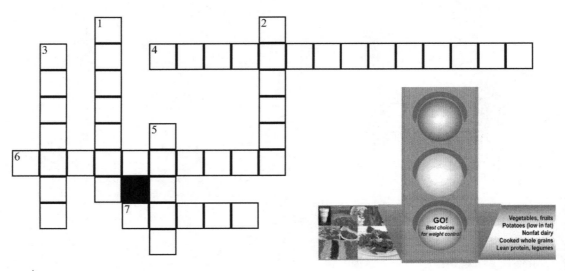

Across:

4. Comparison of foods according to how many calories they contain by a certain weight like ounces or pounds

6. Lettuce, tomatoes, corn, and broccoli are a few foods in this important group

7. Oranges, apples, grapes, and pears are included in this important group.

Down:

1. An important member of the protein family made from dried beans; these are high in fiber and low in calorie density. They should be a part of every good diet.

2. This food group includes pasta, rice, oats, and barley. The lowest-calorie versions are cooked so they are high in moisture. If you pick whole-grain versions, they will be high in fiber, too.

3. This food group includes eggs, poultry, fish, meat, nuts, and seeds. Keep choices lean and low in fat.

5. Skim milk and fat-free yogurt are two examples in this food group that should be kept low in fat and sugar.

Answers: Across: 4. caloriedensity, 6. vegetables, 7. fruits. Down: 1. legumes, 2. grains, 3. protein, 5. dairy.

Healthful Shopping List

Vegetables:
_____ lettuce
_____ spinach
_____ tomatoes
_____ cucumbers
_____ bell peppers
_____ mushrooms
_____ avocado
_____ carrots
_____ celery
_____ broccoli
_____ zucchini
_____ squash
_____ eggplant
_____ kale, collards, etc.
_____ cauliflower
_____ cabbage
_____ corn
_____ herbs _____
_____ onions
_____ garlic
_____ potatoes
_____ tofu
_____ other _____
_____ other _____
_____ other _____
_____ other _____

Fruits:
_____ strawberries
_____ raspberries
_____ blueberries
_____ bananas
_____ apples
_____ pears
_____ peaches
_____ plums
_____ watermelon
_____ cantaloupe
_____ honeydew
_____ pineapple
_____ oranges
_____ grapefruit
_____ lemons/limes
_____ grapes
_____ kiwi
_____ other _____

Packaged:
_____ baked tortilla chips
_____ baked potato chips
_____ whole-grain crackers
　　　 (low in fat)
Cereal:
**(buy whole-grain cereal with >
3 g fiber and < 10 g sugar per
serving)**
_____ shredded wheat
_____ oatmeal
_____ other
Canned:
Vegetables and beans:
**Compare brands to find low-
sodium versions**
**Fruits: Look for items canned
in water or juice, rather than
syrup**
_____ tomatoes
_____ tomato paste
_____ tomato sauce
_____ pasta sauce
_____ hominy
_____ black beans
_____ pinto beans
_____ cannelini beans
_____ garbanzo beans
_____ kidney beans
_____ low-fat soup
_____ chicken broth
_____ canned fruit in juice
_____ unsweetened applesauce
_____ canned vegetables
_____ tuna fish in water
_____ Parmesan cheese
Dried:
_____ beans
_____ lentils
_____ brown rice
_____ macaroni
_____ lasagna
_____ fettucini/linguini
_____ spaghetti
_____ penne
_____ barley
_____ corn meal

_____ raisins
_____ walnuts
_____ almonds
_____ vanilla extract
_____ baking powder
_____ baking soda
_____ cocoa powder
_____ prune puree
_____ peanut butter
_____ herbs _____
_____ spices
_____ vegetable oil
Condiments:
_____ no-salt ketchup
_____ mustard
_____ relish
_____ light soy sauce
_____ balsamic vinegar
_____ vinegar
_____ Worcestershire
_____ low-fat mayo
_____ reduced-calorie syrup
_____ low-fat salad dressing
_____ light jam
_____ light chocolate syrup
Bread:
_____ 100% whole wheat bread
_____ whole-wheat pitas
_____ low-fat tortillas
_____ corn tortilla
Dairy:
_____ fat-free light yogurt
_____ low-fat cheese
_____ skim milk
_____ 100% orange juice
_____ nonfat ricotta cheese
_____ nonfat sour cream
_____ light margarine
_____ fat-free half-n-half

Low-Cal Recipes

Grilled Chicken Pita

   1 Tbsp olive oil
   3 Tbsp balsamic vinegar
1/4 cup fat-free Italian dressing
   1 Tbsp chopped fresh basil
     Black pepper to taste
   4 slices eggplant, 1/2 inch thick
   2 skinless chicken breasts
   2 plum tomatoes, cored and halved
   4 whole wheat pitas, halved

Directions:

1. Preheat the grill or grill pan over medium-high heat.

2. Combine the oil, vinegar, dressing, basil and pepper in a large bowl.

3. Grill the eggplant, chicken and tomatoes until done, brushing with the dressing as you go. Cut each into slices and stuff into the pita halves.

4. Wrap pitas in foil and serve warm, or chill for later use.

Serving idea: This pita can be topped with a little feta cheese. Pitas go well with a tossed salad or grilled corn.

Serves 4. Each serving (2 pita halves): 268 calories, 6 g fat, 1 g saturated fat, 0 g trans fat, 36 mg cholesterol, 528 mg sodium, 27 g carbohydrate, 6.5 g fiber, 21 g protein.

Chicken Pepper Stir-Fry

   1 tablespoon grated ginger
   2 cups stir-fry vegetables
   1 cup broccoli florets
   1 cup red bell pepper strips
   4 Tbsp light soy sauce
   1 Tbsp sesame oil
Granulated garlic to taste
   1 cup cooked white chicken meat, skinless and
     cut into cubes
   3 cups cooked brown rice

Directions:

1. Lightly spray a large, nonstick skillet with vegetable cooking spray and heat it over medium-high heat.

2. Sauté the ginger, vegetables, broccoli, and red peppers until crisp-tender and heated through, about 5 minutes. Season the vegetables with soy sauce and sesame oil and add the chicken, cooking until heated through. Serve the vegetables over rice.

Serves 4. Each serving: 2 cups: 306 calories, 6 g fat, 1 g saturated fat, 0 g trans fat, 29 mg cholesterol, 540 mg sodium, 43 g carbohydrates, 4 g fiber, 20 g protein.

A Salad a Day Keeps the Scale at Bay

There are many reasons to eat a salad. Salads are delicious, healthy, and full of vitamins. Plus, if you want to lose weight, having a salad every day could help you reach your goal.

One of our favorite studies demonstrated that people who eat a low-fat salad before a meal generally consume fewer calories (at that meal) than people who did not have a salad. Take care, however, because the people who loaded their salads with high-fat cheese and dressing actually consumed MORE calories.

Another study indicated that eating acetic acid (which is found in vinegar) may help boost satiety. Satiety is another name for the feeling that you get when you have had enough to eat.

While more research is needed, it is a good idea to eat a salad topped with healthy, low-fat ingredients before a meal. Be sure to include plenty of vinegar. After all, unlike most processed salad dressings, vinegar is naturally fat-free and low in sodium.

Best Toppings

Fresh vegetables, nuts, fruit, dried tomatoes, lemon zest, and chopped hot peppers add flavor, texture, and tons of vitamins. Vinegar, lemon juice, and fat-free dressing are best for those trying to lose weight.

Worst Toppings

Cheese, high-fat dressing, croutons, and bacon bits are all a part of the worst topping list because they contain a fair amount of fat, calories and/or sodium. Use these rarely.

Time-Saving Tips

- Make once, serve twice. Make a large bowl of salad and serve the dressing on the side. That way, you can have the rest again the next day.
- Make it an entrée. Add cooked chicken or fish to your favorite tossed salad and you have an easy and healthful meal.
- Put it in a pita, and you will have a perfect salad to eat on the run.
- For easy recipes, see *www.foodandhealth.com*

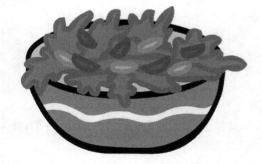

Flavorful vinegars to try include: white wine vinegar, red wine vinegar, balsamic vinegar, rice wine vinegar, cider vinegar and raspberry vinegar.

Skinny Tossed Salad

6 cups ready-to-serve romaine
1/2 cup cucumber, sliced
10 fresh cherry tomatoes, halved
2/3 cup grated carrots
1 teaspoon olive oil
3 tablespoons cider vinegar
Black pepper to taste

Place salad ingredients a large bowl and chill until ready to serve, up to 24 hours. When you're ready, toss the salad with vinegar, a little oil, and pepper. Serve immediately.
Serves 4.

Fruits and Vegetables on the Go

Most Americans do not get enough fruits and vegetables. MyPlate and the Dietary Guidelines for Americans call for most people to eat around 4.5 cups of vegetables and fruits each day.

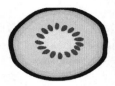

Adding enough fruits and veggies to your diet is one of the most important steps that you can take on the road to good nutrition. Eating enough fruits and vegetables will help you get plenty of vitamins, nutrients, and fiber, which all help you lower your risk for many diseases. Eat fruits and veggies instead of more fattening, high-calorie options

Try fruit for breakfast. One of the quickest combos that you can grab on your way out the door is a banana and 100% juice box. You can also combine fruit with cereal or yogurt. Smoothies are also great for people on the go, just keep them on the small side.

Have a great big salad for lunch. Most places, including McDonalds, offer an entree salad on their menu. Make sure that you are choosing low-calorie ingredients and keeping the dressing low in fat. You can also pack salads and fruits at home and bring them with you.

Have more vegetables with dinner. Try stir-fry dishes, baked potatoes, vegetable soup, vegetarian chili, and pasta with veggies during the week. Another salad or vegetable side dish will help you reach your fruit and veggie goals too.

Don't forget to have fruit for snacks and desserts. Many convenience stores and fast food restaurants carry fruit, and it even travels well from home.

Fruits and vegetables on the go:
- McDonald's - fruit and walnut salad, side salad, apple dippers.
- Starbucks - fruit salad
- Wendy's - baked potato, salad
- Grocery stores - the produce aisle has many convenience packs and salad bars
- Convenience stores - many offer fresh fruits and salads

Easiest to take with you:
- apples
- bananas
- grapes (in bags)
- baby carrots (in bags)
- tangerines
- pears
- canned fruits (packed in juice)

How to pack a salad for lunch:
- Place the lettuce and veggies in a plastic container. Nuts and croutons can go in a baggie on the side.
- Add a small travel container of vinegar or lowfat dressing to your lunchbox. Then you can add it to your meal right before you eat it and things won't get soggy.

What's counts as a cup?
- 2 cups raw leafy greens
- 1 cup fruit or vegetables. They can be canned, fresh, frozen, raw, or cooked.
- 1/2 cup dried fruit
- 1 cup 100% fruit or vegetable juice

Portion Control

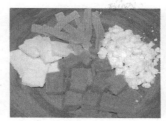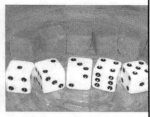

It is easy to eat too much cheese – a one-ounce portion is 5 cubes, about the size of 5 dice.

How can you deal with oversized servings? It can be hard to stop eating when there is tons of delicious food to enjoy.

A common answer to the problem is to ignore the rest of the food and only eat proper portions of each item. Sadly, that can be difficult.

First of all, studies show that when people are offered larger portions of food, they tend to eat more calories. In one study, participants ate 30% more calories when offered the largest portion of an entrée, compared to what they ate when they were offered the smallest portion (Am J Clin Nutr 2002;76(6):1207-1213). When there is lots of food on your plate, it can skew your perception of what you've eaten and make it hard to stop eating.

Second, even when you pay attention to portion size, you also have to consider WHAT you are eating. Even small portions of high-fat, high-calorie foods can interfere with the best weight loss plans.

Take a look at the chart below. It demonstrates that guessing is no substitute for properly measuring servings. Take the time to become aware of how much you are eating. Start with measuring cups and spoons to make sure you're on track.

Avoid Pitfalls of Oversized Servings

- Eating out of the bag - This makes it very easy to eat much more than one serving without realizing it.

- Pouring tons of dressing on your salad - Dressing is often calorie dense. Try pouring just a few capfuls instead.

- Using an oversized bowl - This mistake occurred on our cereal and ice cream tests. Use smaller bowls to serve food and start measuring the portions you put into those bowls.

- Slathering enough butter or margarine to really cover the whole slice of bread - Think about the size of your thumbtip and use that much or less when spreading butter or margarine on bread.

Serving Size Test Results

Our test staff guessed about proper serving sizes using the foods listed below. Their guesses for a single portion were often much more than one serving! Follow the tips on the right so that you can use actual serving sizes with these common foods.

Item	Guess	Actual portion	Tip for better portion control
Cereal	3 cups	1 cup	Use smaller bowl and measuring cup
Cheese	3 ounces	1 ounce	Picture 5 dice for a one-ounce portion
Meat/poultry	9 ounces	3 ounces	Visualize a deck of cards for one serving
Bagged snacks	3-5 ounces	1 ounce	One or two handfuls
Salad dressing	3-4 ounces	2 tablespoons	2 capfuls
Ice cream	3 cups	1/2 cup	Half-cup scoop; smaller glass; add fruit
Butter	1 tablespoon	1 teaspoon	Use the tip of your thumb as a guide

The Dietary Guidelines for Americans explain, "Portion Size [is] the amount of a food consumed in one eating occasion."

Examine the Facts

Follow 3 easy steps for healthful food choices

1. **Look at serving size, servings per container, and calories.**

2. **Limit fat, saturated fat, trans fat, cholesterol, and sodium.**

3. **Get enough fiber and important nutrients.**

Eating too many calories per day is linked to obesity and the development of certain chronic diseases.

Eating too much fat, saturated fat, trans fat, cholesterol, or sodium may increase your risk for certain diseases.

Eating enough fiber and nutrients can improve your health and reduce your risk of some diseases.

Nutrition Facts

Serving Size 1/4 cup (36g)
Serving Per Container: 9

Amount per serving

Calories 60   Calories from Fat 0

	% Daily Value
Total Fat 0g	0%
Saturated Fat 0g	0%
Trans Fat 0g	
Cholesterol 0mg	0%
Sodium 15mg	1%
Total Carbohydrate 22g	7%
Dietary Fiber 14g	56%
Sugars 1g	
Protein 7g	

Vitamin A 0%		Vitamin C 0%	
Calcium 4%		Iron	15%

Daily Value – how a food fits into a daily plan:

- 5% or less is low

- 20% or more is high

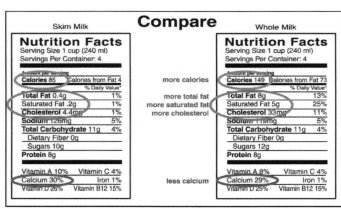

Skim Milk	Compare	Whole Milk

Nutrition Facts — Skim Milk
Serving Size 1 cup (240 ml)
Servings Per Container: 4

Amount per serving
Calories 85   Calories from Fat 4

	% Daily Value*
Total Fat 0.4g	1%
Saturated Fat .2g	1%
Cholesterol 4.4mg	1%
Sodium 126mg	5%
Total Carbohydrate 11g	4%
Dietary Fiber 0g	
Sugars 10g	
Protein 8g	
Vitamin A 10% Vitamin C 4%	
Calcium 30% Iron 1%	
Vitamin D 26% Vitamin B12 15%	

more calories
more total fat
more saturated fat
more cholesterol
less calcium

Nutrition Facts — Whole Milk
Serving Size 1 cup (240 ml)
Servings Per Container: 4

Amount per serving
Calories 149   Calories from Fat 73

	% Daily Value*
Total Fat 8g	13%
Saturated Fat 5g	25%
Cholesterol 33mg	11%
Sodium 119mg	5%
Total Carbohydrate 11g	4%
Dietary Fiber 0g	
Sugars 12g	
Protein 8g	
Vitamin A 8% Vitamin C 4%	
Calcium 29% Iron 1%	
Vitamin D 25% Vitamin B12 15%	

Daily Dietary Goals:

- Total fat	20-35% calories
- Saturated fat	Less than 10% calories
- Trans fat	Less than 1% calories
- Cholesterol	Less than 300 mg
- Sodium	Less than 2,300 mg*
- Total carbohydrate	45-65% calories
- Dietary fiber	14g per 1,000 calories
- Protein	10-35% calories

For personal eating programs, visit choosemyplate.gov

* Limit sodium to 1,500 mg per day if you have hypertension or are at risk for getting it.

Portions Are Larger Now

Look At the Difference

	20 Yrs Ago	Today
Cheeseburger	333	590
French fries	210	610
Soda	85	250
Turkey sandwich	320	820
Popcorn	270	630
Cheesecake	260	640
Cookie	55	275
Coffee	45	350
Muffin	210	500
Pizza	500	850
TOTAL CALORIES	2288	5655

Source: US Dept of Health and Human Services

The photo above is part of a summary of information from the US Department of Health and Human Services, the National Institute of Health, and the National Heart Lung and Blood Institute. The point? Portion sizes have grown over the past 20 years.

Take a look at the total calories in each column. If you ate everything on that picture 20 years ago, you would consume 2,288 calories. Today, if you ate the same foods, you would consume 5,655 calories.

According to a study in the *Journal of the American Medical Association*, between 1977 and 1996, salty snacks, desserts, soft drinks, burgers, and French fries have all markedly increased in size and calories. They're still increasing today.

In restaurants, portions are out of control. Between super sizes, all-you-can-eat buffets, and huge platters of food delivered to the table, how is a person supposed to eat a reasonable, balanced meal? Even grocery stores and wholesale clubs want you to "buy more and save more."

Meanwhile, at home, plates and bowls are getting bigger. Plus, there's plenty of room in our refrigerators, freezers, and pantries to store bargain-sized packages of foods.

Could all this be linked to the growing rate of obesity in the U.S.? Think about it… larger serving sizes mean more calories. Weight gain is caused by taking in more calories than you burn. We believe that out-of-control serving sizes lead to out-of-control weight!

For More Information

http://www.nhlbi.nih.gov/ - Search for Portion Distortion, take the quiz, and review the facts.

http://www.cdc.gov - "Portion Size Pitfalls" is a multi-page handout that can be turned into a board game. Try it out and see for yourself! Just search the site for "portion control."

Use Your Plate to Eat Right

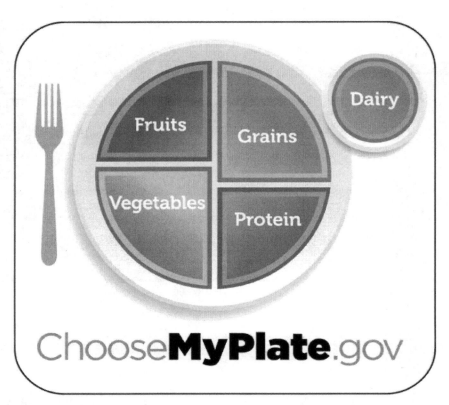

MyPlate Rocks the House

Build your plate as the mirror image to MyPlate whenever possible. Fill half with fruits and veggies, and divide up lowfat dairy, grains, and protein for the rest. Be sure to follow more of MyPlate's advice and keep portions small. Stick to lowfat, low sugar dairy when possible, and make at least half the grains you eat whole grains. It is also wise to eat a variety of protein foods, not just chicken or beef.

MyPlate offers great ways to control portins and eat balanced meals. Check out *www.choose-myplate.gov* for a personalized eating plan and even more strategies for crafting healthy meals.

The Great Plate Switch

It also helps to start using smaller plates at home. Make a salad on a dinner plate and serve dinner on a salad plate! This strategy will help save you calories and add extra nutrients.

Sharing is Caring

- Share an entrée with a friend.
- Split your meal in half and put the other half in a doggie bag for another meal.
- Order soup AND salad, but nothing else.

Other Ways to Downsize Eating Out...

- Skip the bread basket.
- Order appetizer portions as entrees. Oh, and no, this does not apply to appetizer samplers that should be shared by multiple people.
- Order the smallest size at the drive-thru or research the meal's calorie count online before you even get in the car.

Take Portion Control on a Road Trip

Practice eyeballing proper portions at home. Check your work with measuring cups and spoons until you have become a portion control master. This will help you evaluate restaurant servings.

Big + Baked = Diet Mistake

Look at the Size of Your Treats!

Baked goods can be calorie bombs, especially since their portions seem to be getting more and more out of control.

Most baked goods sold in coffee shops are HUGE. Unfortunately, the calories they contain match their size. For example, if you ate one of everything listed in the Starbucks nutritional guide, you would consume over 32,000 calories. That sounds like a lot, but you would only need to eat one item a day for 80 days to get to that amount of calories! Everyday decisions can have a great impact on your waist over time.

Most bagels, cookies, brownies, bars, muffins and cakes offered in restaurants and coffee stores are upwards of 400 calories each.

So what's the solution?

Buy small! Take a look at the items on the bottom chart. They are smaller and contain far fewer calories than their counterparts in the top chart.

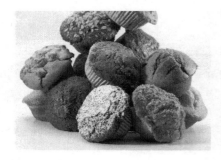

Starbucks Fresh Baked Goods	Size (g)	Cals	Fat
Caramel Pecan Sticky Roll	184	730	40
Chocolate Peanut Butter Stack	142	670	42
Crumb Cake	163	670	32
Cinnamon Roll	170	620	29
Seven Layer Bar	133	600	37
Caramel Brownie	126	580	36
Classic Coffee Cake	139	570	28
Iced Carrot Pound Cake	177	540	13
Butterscotch Pecan Scone	120	520	27
Chocolate Marshmallow Bar	113	510	27
Cinnamon Chip Scone with Icing	128	510	23
Iced Lemon Pound Cake	142	500	23
Maple Oat Scone with Icing	128	490	22
Orange Poppy Pound Cake	122	490	27
Pecan Diamond	86	490	37
Holiday Gingerbread	126	480	16
White Chocolate Macadamia Nut Cookie	99	470	27
Blueberry Scone	128	460	18
Cheese Danish with Mocha Swirls	120	460	28

Dark Chocolate Graham	28	140	8
Milk Chocolate Graham	28	140	8
Chocolate Hazelnut Biscotti	28	110	5
Vanilla Almond Biscotti	28	110	5
Shortbread	20	100	6
Madeline	17	80	3.5
Crisp Cinnamon Twist	13	60	2

Case Study: Overeating Healthy Foods

Even healthy calories can cause weight gain if you eat too many of them. That's why it's so important to use portion control.

Meet PortionDistorter

Height	5'4"
Weight	162
BMI	28
BMI category	Overweight
Waist Circumference	37"

Notes:

PortionDistorter presented to a registered dietitian (RD) with an interest in weight loss. Her medical history was excellent, but her last annual check-up revealed a slight elevation in triglyceride levels. PortionDistorter had always been active and never had to worry about her weight. She is an avid exerciser with a weekly routine of cardio and weight training. She works out for 45 minutes to 1 hour at least 5 times per week. She also runs 5k and 10k races for fun and walks everywhere. She recently started dating a man who enjoys running with her, but likes taking her out to restaurants too.

Upon nutrition assessment, PortionDistorter proclaimed herself a "health nut" and listed the types of foods she eats on a daily basis. Additionally, she turned in a 7-day food log. When asked what her weight loss goal was, she stated a somewhat lofty goal of 25 lb within 2 months so she could look good for her 10-year high school reunion.

PortionDistorter's diet sounded healthy, and her exercise plan seems great. So what was the problem? What did her food log reveal?

Nutrition Assessment:

Upon examining the composition of PortionDistorter's diet, the RD realized that PortionDistorter is choosing high-fiber whole grains, lean sources of protein, "good" fats, and adding vegetables to meals. For the most part, she is only drinking water with and between meals (7 – 8 oz glasses per day). However, the RD was also able to identify the secret to PortionDistorter's weight gain. The an lay in the amount of total food consumed (calories in) versus calories out. The equation was not balanced, and PortionDistorter was taking in many more calories than she burned off.

PortionDistorter's Food Log - Example Day

Breakfast   6:00 AM   890 calories

1 whole wheat bagel with 2 tablespoons of peanut butter, 8 oz. fruit-flavored yogurt, 8 oz. orange juice

Lunch   1: 30 PM   700 calories

Panera tuna salad sandwich on honey wheat bread, 16 oz. water

Snack   4:30 PM   680 calories

1 cup trail mix (½ c. almonds + ½ c. raisins), water

Dinner   8:30 PM   750 calories

2 cups brown rice, 3 oz. roasted chicken breast (without skin), 1 cup steamed broccoli with a tablespoon of olive oil and fresh garlic, water

Snack   10:30 PM   180 calories

1 Kashi Go-Lean bar, water

Total Calories In = 3200

Calories Out (energy expenditure)

2 miles walking to/from work (~20 minutes), 35 minutes on elliptical machine at high intensity, 20 minutes of stretching

Total Calories Out = 705

3200 – 705 = Total Calories 2495

Food Log Makeover

Nutrition Recommendations:

1. Set realistic goals: The RD explained that losing 25 pounds in 8 weeks was not realistic. For long-term weight loss, losing 1 lb per week is recommended. The RD told PortionDistorter that if she ate 500 fewer calories every day (3,500 calories per week), she would be within healthy limits and probably be more successful in the long run.

2. Keep daily food logs: Include calorie counts. Did you know that the average American underestimates daily caloric intake by over 600 calories per day (Tufts University Health & Wellness Letter, 2004)? However, when you write down what you eat every day, it increases awareness of portion size, quality of food, timing of meals/snacks, and hunger/fullness cues.

3. Eat high fiber, low fat meals & snacks. The RD suggested that PortionDistorter set calorie limits at 1800 calories/day. She further broke it down into 350 calories at breakfast, 550 calories at lunch, 600 calories at dinner, and 300 calories divded into 2 snacks per day. The RD also recommended getting 25 -30 grams of fiber per day. Not only does fiber put off hunger by improving fullness, it also significantly lowers cholesterol levels.

4. Follow MyPlate: It's easy to pay attention to portion size when a plate is set up to look like MyPlate. Ideally, half the plate should be filled with colorful vegetables and fruits. Stick to small portions of lean protein, whole grains, and lowfat dairy to round out the meal.

5. Eat every 4 to 5 hours.

PortionDistorter should rev up her metabolism by eating less food, more frequently. She was told not to go longer than 5 hours without a meal. The best method to keep metabolism humming throughout the day is to supply the body with small doses of fuel at regular intervals. This will stop it from slowing into "starvation" mode. Think of metabolism as a fire that has to be fed/adjusted every 3-4 hours in order to keep burning fuel efficiently.

Outcome:

Within 6 months of working with the RD, PortionDistorter lost 16 pounds (~10% of her body weight). Her Body Mass Index dropped to 25, which is within the healthy range, and her waist shrunk from 37 inches to 34 inches. Over time, PortionDistorter learned how to adjust portion sizes for all foods. Her snacks were kept to 100 – 150 calories and she was conscious about not going too long without eating. Her energy levels improved and she even felt better while working out.

Food Log Makeover for PortionDistorter

Breakfast   6:00 AM   310 calories

1 cup Kashi whole grain cereal, 8 oz skim milk, 1 medium apple

Snack   9:00 AM   180 calories

4 oz. cottage cheese, 2 Tbsp. raisins, water

Lunch   12:30 PM   565 calories

3 oz. turkey breast, 2 slices Natural Ovens whole grain bread, 1 slice tomato, lettuce, 1 Tbsp. mustard, ½ cup baby carrots, 8 oz low-fat yogurt, 3-4 whole almonds, water

Snack   4:00 PM   135 calories

1 tbsp peanut butter, 2 Wasa high-fiber crackers, water

Dinner   8:00 PM   600 calories

1 cup whole wheat pasta, ½ c tomato sauce, 3 oz. chicken breast, 1 cup broccoli, 1 Tbsp Parmesan cheese, 5 oz wine, water

Total Calories In = 1790   (~815 calories deficit = - 1 ½ lb/week)

Exercise: The Key to Weight Control

Cleaning the bathroom burns way more calories than watching TV. In fact, most light household chores burn twice as many calories as simply sitting still.

This chart highlights the different activities you can do and how many calories you will burn while doing them. Take a look at the differences between sedentary, moderate, and seriously active tasks, then make a pact with yourself to sit less and move more!

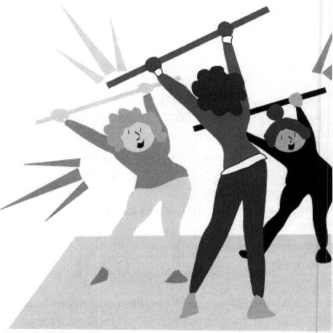

Activity:	Calories Burned Per 30 Minutes:
Sedentary	
Watching TV, computer	38
Moderate activity	
Laundry, folding clothes	76
Making the bed	76
Preparing dinner	78
Washing dishes	81
Vacuuming, sweeping	90
Walking (slowly)	110
Grocery shopping	129
Cleaning the bathroom	129
Washing the car	163
Gardening	172
Very active	
Working out at the gym	200
Yoga	210
Walking (briskly)	211
Aerobics	215
Soccer	250
Spinning	254
Swimming	321
Jogging	360
Kickboxing	384

How Often?

You should do the following on most days in order to reach your goals. Just match what you hope to get out of exercise to the times provided.

30 minutes – to prevent chronic disease

60 minutes – to prevent weight gain

60-90 minutes – to sustain weight loss

Setting aside 30 to 60 minutes each day for planned exercise is one way to make room for physical activity, but it is not the only way. Physical activity can add up over the course of teh day. For example, try exercising for three to six 10-minute sessions before and after school.

Take a look at the example below to see how easy it is to fit 60 minutes of moderate activity in your day:

Cleaning your room	**10 minutes**
Walking briskly after school	**10 minutes**
Helping cook dinner	**10 minutes**
Exercising with a video	**30 minutes**

Success Tips

Just 100 extra calories per day can cause a weight gain of 10 pounds per year! For every 3,500 extra calories you consume, you will gain one pound.

Exercise is a great way to help you burn more calories and guard against storing excess calories as body fat. It also contributes to physical fitness and health.

Any movement (along with the daily living functions of your body) will burn calories. It is only when you burn more calories than you eat or drink that you will lose weight.

Start Slow

Start slow and vary your activities. Beginning too fast will dramatically increase your risk of injury or burnout.

If you have been sedentary for a long time, you should just walk for a few minutes per day at an easy pace. Talk with your doctor to make sure that you are physically able to start an exercise routine. This is especially important if you are new to exercise, have diabetes, have heart disease, or are dealing with any other health issue that may require special care.

Add to It

Think of ways to add to activities that you are already doing. Can you take a walk during lunch? Park farther away? Hand deliver messages? Clean your house more frequently? Walk or go for a run with your friends?

For some families, putting exercise equipment in front of the TV is a big help. We recommend any of the following...

- Stationary bike
- Treadmill
- Stair-climber
- Mat (or calisthenics)
- Exercise ball, resistance bands, or weights

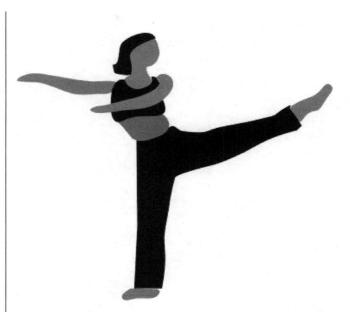

Put on your workout clothes when it is time to work out. Do it before you can talk yourself out of getting started. Even if you can't work out at a planned time, if you're fully prepared, you may be able to fit it in later.

Find a Friend

It helps to have a workout buddy. You are not as likely to skip out on your exercise plans if you know you have someone waiting on you.

Maybe you have a friend at school who can walk with you at lunch? Or a neighbor that likes to go for a run on the weekends? Think about people who might be willing to exercise with you.

Get Active

Visit *www.active.com* and take a look at the walking and sporting events in your area. The site features everything from charity walks to bike rides, 5ks, 10ks, marathons – even triathlons.

It All Adds Up

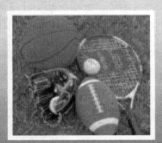

Easy Ways to 60 Minutes

- **Walking briskly before work – 15 minutes**
- **Yardwork – 15 minutes**
- **Lifting weights at gym – 30 minutes**

It all adds up!

As you put together your exercise plan, keep your eyes on the prize. In this case, the prize is the total minutes of accumulated activity each day. Just because you didn't complete an exercise all at once does not mean that your efforts didn't count. If you're facing a busy schedule, break up your activities and do them in little bursts throughout the day.

Some examples include:
- Walking briskly before school — 15 minutes
- Yardwork — 15 minutes
- Gym class — 30 minutes
- Walking at lunch —- 20 minutes
- Walking the dog after dinner — 15 minutes

Variety and consistency are the keys to a solid exercise routine. Keep things fresh and stick to your exercise goals. If something gets boring, change it. Don't give it up without a replacement.

Researchers at Maastricht University in the Netherlands concluded that people who engage in moderate physical activity had the highest overall physical activity levels.

Their study of 30 men and women over a two-week period also revealed that those who exercised vigorously for short periods of time compensated for that activity by spending a greater part of their day sitting or lying down.

Sure, vigorous exercise burns more calories, but the moderate exercisers tended to be more active overall. (Source: *Nature* 2001; 410, 539).

For more information, visit the Center for Disease Control online at www.cdc.gov.

Try a Pedometer to Measure Activity

Use a Pedometer to Measure Activity

It all adds up!

- 2,500 steps = average person/day
- 8,000 steps = 1 extra mile = 100 calories
- 10,000 steps = 2 extra miles = 200 calories
- 12,000 steps= 3 extra miles = 300 calories

A useful tool to measure activity is a pedometer. A pedometer measures not only how much planned exercise a person gets, but also how active that person is throughout the day.

Where to start

The average person typically takes about 2,500 steps per day, just going about their daily activities. 2,500 steps usually covers just over one mile.

If you can increase your steps to 8,000 per day, you will have traveled the equivalent of 4 miles.

Taking 10,000 steps per day is what makes a difference in your efforts to lose weight. Don't worry, it's not as hard as you might think.

Try taking 10,000 steps in a single day and see how you do. Once you've mastered that, see if you can reach 10,000 by noon. Challenge yourself to increase and improve!

How to wear a pedometer

You will need to wear the pedometer above your hip bone. Hook it to your belt or waist band. Do not put it in your pocket because it won't register properly. Plus, you might lose it. A pedometer leash is great because it keeps the pedometer from falling off.

How to purchase a pedometer

Good quality, accurate pedometers usually cost around $25. Look in sporting goods and fitness stores in your area or do a search online.

For more information

For more information see *smallstep.gov*. This site has health tips, activitiy trackers, links to local resources and inspirational stories to help you stay motivated.

Exercise Log

Online calorie calculators:
www.caloriecontrol.org

Find out more at:
www.health.gov

Date   **Time**   **Activity (or Number of Steps)**

_____

_____

_____

_____

_____

_____

_____

_____

_____

_____

_____

_____

_____

_____

_____

_____

_____

_____

_____

_____

_____

_____

_____

_____

_____

_____

_____

_____

_____

_____

Beverage Calories: Are They Going to Waist?

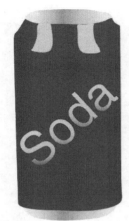

The Dietary Guidelines for Americans advise us to limit the added sugars we eat and drink. After all, almost half of all the added sugars in the average American's diet come from soda and other sugary drinks.[1]

According to research published in the *International Journal of Obesity*, calories from liquids like sodas, sports beverages, or sweetened teas don't seem to register as food to the people who drink them.[2]

Participants in a study at Purdue University were asked to eat 450 calories worth of jelly beans every day for four weeks and to drink 450 calories worth of soda every day for another four weeks.

On days that they ate the jelly beans, the participants ate roughly 450 fewer calories of other foods. Therefore, they ate no more calories than usual.

But on days that they drank the soda, the participants didn't compensate at all. They ended up eating roughly 450 more calories than usual.

Be aware of how many sweetened drinks you are drinking during the day. Try to make adjustments so you are enjoying calorie-free beverages. Remember, MyPlate advises people to replace sugary drinks with water.

Be aware of portion sizes, which can be larger than you might expect. A king-sized soda at Burger King has 35 ounces. That's just over one quart! 7-Eleven features a "Slurp and Gulp" combo drink that has a total of 54 ounces of soda/slurpee. That's almost 7 cups of that sugary mix! Furthermore, many restaurants and movie theaters offer unlimited refills, which can really add up without being obvious.

Take a look at the dangers of too many liquid calories.

Calories:

8 oz of orange juice	120
24 oz of soda	292
Grand total:	**412**

References:

1) *JADA*, 2000.
2) *International Journal of Obesity*, June 2000, 24(6):794-800.
3) Dietary Reference Intakes for Water, Potassium, Sodium, Chloride, and Sulfate (2004)

Tips for Beverages:

1) Eat whole fruit instead of drinking fruit juice. This will make you feel more full and add fiber to your diet too.

2) Switch to calorie-free sodas, like sparkling water with a twist of lime or lemon.

3) Most people need to drink about a gallon of water per day depending on climate and their physical activity levels.

4) Flavor coffee and tea with skim milk or fat-free half and half. Use low-calorie sugar substitutes such as Splenda®, Equal®, or NutraSweet®. Keep in mind that just a teaspoon of full-fat creamer and a tablespoon of sugar have 45 calories each. This adds 90 additional calories to the drink. If a person adds a each measurement to a daily cup of coffee, that person could consume an additional 32,850 calories in a year.

By Victoria Shanta-Retelny, RD, LD.

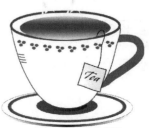

Where Do Added Sugars Come From?

Quiz: What is the primary source of added sugar in the American Diet?

1. Soda, fruit drinks

2. Sugars and candy

3. Cakes, cookies, and pies

4. Dairy desserts and milk products

5. Other grain foods

ANSWER: #1. Sugary drinks are the single biggest source of refined sugars in the American diet. Together, these drinks make up 43% of all the added sugars that Americans eat or drink.

Added sugars are sugars and syrups that are added to foods or beverages during processing or preparation. They are not naturally-occurring sugars like those that you might find in milk and fruit.

Source: *American Journal of Clinical Nutrition* 1995: 62 (suppl): 178S-194S.

Quiz: One can of soda contains about 40 grams of sugar. How many teaspoons is this?

1. 40

2. 4

3. 10

4. 20

5. 8

ANSWER: 10 teaspoons! That is almost the same amount of sugar that is in a 2-ounce bag of Skittles. Refined sugar contributes only empty calories and no nutrients at all.

The phrase, "empty calories" describes the content of high-energy foods with poor nutritional profiles. An empty calorie has the same energy content of any other calorie but lacks accompanying nutrients and fiber.

Source: Michael Jacobson, head of the Center for Science in the Public Interest, coined the term in 1972.

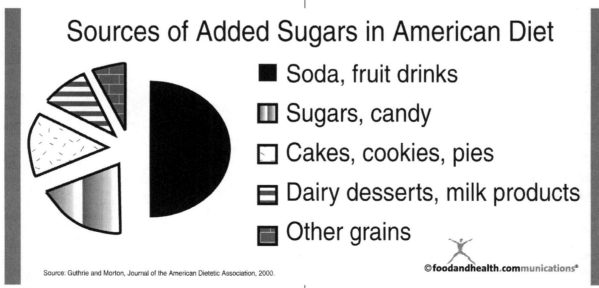

Sources of Added Sugars in American Diet

- Soda, fruit drinks
- Sugars, candy
- Cakes, cookies, pies
- Dairy desserts, milk products
- Other grains

Source: Guthrie and Morton, Journal of the American Dietetic Association, 2000.

©foodandhealth.communications®

Each year, Americans consume an average of more than 52 gallons of soft drinks per person.

Are You Beverage Smart?

High-Cal:

Chocolate shake, 16 oz	580
Creamy coffee drink, 16 oz	480
Large smoothie, 22 oz	354
Soda, 32 oz	310
Juice drink, 21 oz	250
Sport drink, 32 oz	200
Tea (sweet), 20 oz bottle	175

Low-Cal:

Coffee*, 16 oz	10
Diet tea, 20 oz	0
Water, 16 oz	0
Brewed tea*, 16 oz	0
Diet soda, 16 oz	0

*No sugar added

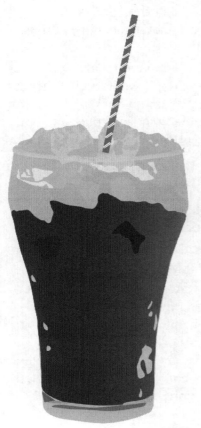

_____ Are you getting enough water?

Daily water intake must be balanced with losses in order to maintain proper hydration.

Most people need to drink about a gallon per day, depending on the climate and their physical activity levels.

_____ Do you limit the amount of sweetened beverages you consume?

The Dietary Guidelines for Americans insist, "Beverages with caloric sweeteners, sugars and sweets, and other sweetened foods that provide little or no nutrients are negatively associated with diet quality and can contribute to excessive energy intakes."

_____ Do you limit the fat in your drinks?

Switch to low-fat or skim milk. Remember, MyPlate advises people to choose lowfat options whenever they're considering dairy foods. Limit the amount and sizes of shakes you consume, and be aware of what you add to your cup of coffee or tea.

For more information:
- _www.health.gov/DietaryGuidelines_
- _www.starbucks.com_
- _www.mcdonalds.com_
- _www.jambajuice.com_
- _www.planetsmoothie.com_
- _www.gatorade.com_

5 Ways to Lower Beverage Calories

1. Make better coffee choices.

Some beverages pack as many calories as a meal! Watch out for options that are high in fat and sugar, like the ones listed here...

	Calories:
Coffee Coolatta® with Cream	*350*
Mocha swirl latte	*230*
Coffee with cream and sugar	*120*

There are strategies that you can use to make your coffee drinks healthier. We've collected our favorites below...

- Order coffee drinks that are made with skim milk.
- Try herbal tea.
- Try drinking your drink without sweeteners.

Iced latte with skim milk	*70*
Coffee with skim milk	*25*
Plain coffee	*10*

If you drink coffee every day, and would replace cream and sugar with non-nutritive sweetener, you would save almost 35,000 calories over the course of a year. That's about 10 pounds!

2. Choose whole fruit instead of smoothies or juice.

While most blended drinks do contain fruit, they also often include frozen yogurt, sherbet, cream, and/or added sugar, all of which add calories. Plus, many of the regular sized cups at smoothie shops can fit more than three cups of smoothie inside. That comes to about 500 calories per container!

It is best to eat whole fruit instead of fruit juice or smoothies. Whole fruit packs more fiber, which will keep you feeling full for a longer period of time than fruit juice would. The fiber that fruit contains also helps lower your cholesterol.

3. Shrink your sodas

Super-sized or extra-large beverages may be a bargain per ounce, but they are a disaster for your waistline. Compare:

Large cola (32 ounce)	*310 calories*
Small cola (16 ounce)	*150 calories*

310 or 150 calories may not sound like much, but, over time, this can make a big impact! 310 multiplied by 365 days is 113,149 calories or 32 pounds per year and 150 calories multiplied by 365 is 54,750 or 15 pounds per year.

Did you know that a "child-sized" soda in a fast food restaurant contains the same amount of liquid as a 12-ounce can?

4. Drink skim milk instead of whole milk.

An eight-ounce serving of whole milk contains 160 calories. The same-size serving of skim milk contains just half as many calories!

Limit the number of shakes you consume. If you don't want to give them up entirely, try making your own small versions at home with skim milk and real fruit. Frozen fruit makes a shake thick and cold!

5. Make the best choices for every day.

Water, 16 oz	0
Brewed tea, 16 oz	0
Diet soda, 16 oz	0
Diet tea, 20 oz	0

Stock the fridge with grab-and-go bottles of water and low-calorie beverages. Having the right foods and beverages on hand is a key to controlling your calories. This helps keep you from making a bad "on the run" choice when away from home. Remember, MyPlate advises people to replace sugary drinks with water.

Discretionary Calories

What are discretionary calories?

Y ou need a certain number of calories to keep up your energy levels, for physical activity, and to help your body function. Think of the calories that you need for energy like money you have to spend. Each person has a total calorie "budget." This budget can be divided into two categories: essentials and extras.

With a financial budget, the essentials are items like rent and food. The extras are more like movie tickets and vacations.

In a calorie budget, the "essentials" are the minimum calories required to meet your nutrient needs. By choosing the lowest fat and no-sugar-added forms of foods in each food group from MyPlate, you would make the best nutrient choices.

Depending on the foods you choose, you may be able to spend more calories than the amount required to meet your nutrient needs. These calories are the "extras" that can be used on luxuries like solid fats and added sugars, or on more food from any food group. They are your discretionary calories.

Each person has an allowance for some discretionary calories. Many people have used up this allowance before lunch!

Most discretionary calorie allowances are very small. Think between 100 and 300 calories... total. Discretionary calorie budgets are extra small for people who are not physically active. For many, the discretionary calorie allowance is completely used up by the foods they choose in each food group, such as higher fat meats, cheeses, whole milk, or sweetened bakery products.

You can use your discretionary calorie allowance to:

- eat more foods from any food group that MyPlate recommends.

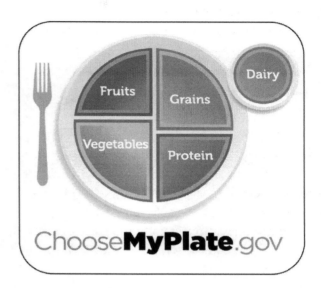

- eat higher calorie forms of foods—those that contain solid fats or added sugars. Examples are whole milk, cheese, sausage, biscuits, sweetened cereal, and sweetened yogurt.

- add fats or sweeteners to foods. Examples include sauces, salad dressings, sugar, syrup, and butter.

- eat or drink items that are mostly fats or caloric sweeteners, such as candy and soda.

For example, assume that your calorie budget is 2,000 calories per day. Of these calories, you need to spend at least 1,735 calories in order to get the essential nutrients your body needs.

This means you have about 265 discretionary calories left. You may use these on "luxury" versions of the foods in each group, such as higher-fat meat or sweetened cereal. Or you can spend them on sweets, sauces, or beverages. Many people overspend their discretionary calorie allowances, choosing more added fats and sugars than their budget allows.

For More Information:
www.choosemyplate.gov

Beverage Recipes

Banana Smoothie

1 cup skim milk

1 banana

1/4 teaspoon ground cinnamon

1/8 teaspoon ground nutmeg

1 tablespoon fat-free whipped cream

Place milk, banana, and spices in a blender and blend on high speed until smooth. Top with whipped cream and enjoy!

Servings: Serves 1, Each serving: 1 cup: 98 calories, 0.7 g fat, 0.5 g saturated fat, 0 g trans fat, 0 mg cholesterol, 56 mg sodium, 19.7 g carbohydrates, 1.5 g dietary fiber, 13 g sugars, 5 g protein.

Diabetic Exchanges:

Fruit: 2.0

Milk: 1.0

Total Preparation & Cooking Time: 5 minutes (5 Prep, 0 Cook)

Fat-Free Latte

1/2 cup brewed decaffeinated coffee (strong)

1/2 cup skim milk

Heat milk in the microwave for 60 to 90 seconds. Add coffee and mix well.

Servings: Serves 1. Each serving: 1 cup: 47 calories, 0.3 g fat, 0 g saturated fat, 0 g trans fat, 2 mg cholesterol, 67 mg sodium, 6.6 g carbohydrate, 0 g fiber, 5.4 g sugars, 4.5 g protein.

Diabetic Exchanges:

Milk: 0.5

Total Preparation & Cooking Time: 4 minutes (2 Prep, 2 Cook)

Minted Green Tea

1 cup boiling water

1 green tea bag

1 sprig fresh mint

Directions:

Place the tea bag and mint in a mug. Pour boiling water into the mug. Allow to steep for 1-2 minutes. Remove the tea bag and serve hot.

Servings: Serves 1. Each serving: 1 cup: 2 calories, 0 g fat, 0 g saturated fat, 0 g trans fat, 0 mg cholesterol, 7 mg sodium, 0 g carbohydrate, 0 g fiber, 0 g sugars, 0 g protein.

Total Preparation & Cooking Time: 4 minutes (2 Prep, 2 Cook)

Spiced Tea Latte

1 cup skim milk

A pinch of each: cinnamon, allspice, cloves

1/2 tsp sugar

1 bag of black tea

Directions:

Place milk, spices, and sugar together in a coffee mug and stir well. Add the tea bag and microwave on medium power until hot, about 2 minutes. Allow to steep for a few minutes, discard tea bag, and serve.

Servings: Serves 1, Each serving 1 cup: 86 calories, 0.4 g fat, 0 g saturated fat, 0 g trans fat, 4 mg cholesterol, 116 mg sodium, 13 g carbohydrate, 0 g fiber, 12 g sugars, 7 g protein.

Total Preparation & Cooking Time: 7 minutes (2 Prep, 5 Cook)

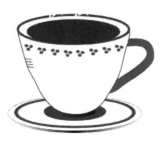

Case Study: Liquid Calorie Sabotage

Meet BeverageSipper:

Height	5'8"
Weight	170
BMI	26
BMI category	Overweight
Waist Circumference	34"

Notes:

BeverageSipper presented to a registered dietitian (RD) at her physician's recommendation. Her medical history was stable, but over the last five years, BeverageSipper's total cholesterol has been climbing and her fasting blood sugar has gone up. She has been experiencing night sweats, unusually frequent cravings for sweets, and recent weight shifting from her hips to her abdominal area. She never had to "watch" what she ate or drank in the past.

Upon nutrition assessment, the RD noted that BeverageSipper has a hard time recalling her food intake. She especially could not remember drinking much. After some thought, she could recite what she consumed in a typical day. For some reason, BeverageSipper did not consider beverages a part of her daily calorie scheme, and, unsurprisingly, it turned out that she drank more than she thought she did. BeverageSipper always drank with meals and never drank diet beverages because she didn't like the taste of sugar substitutes. She was trying to increase her dietary fiber (because she was aware of her cholesterol levels) and had just started to work with a personal trainer on strength training. She also takes daily one hour walks.

What did BeverageSipper's food logs reveal? Although her food intake seemed fairly healthy, her liquid calories really stacked up. In fact, half of the calories she consumed came from the beverages she drank. It soon became apparent that BeverageSipper didn't realize that she was drinking a meal's worth of calories in addtion to her actual meals.

Nutrition Assessment:

Upon examination of the composition of BeverageSipper's diet, the RD noticed that the majority of BeverageSipper's calories were coming from high-calorie beverages. Although she was drinking a lot, she was dehydrated because of the caffeine that most of her beverages contained. Also, she was only drinking two 8 ounce glasses of water per day. The main problem was that BeverageSipper was not conscious of what she was drinking. However, she was already on the road to healthier food and exercise choices.

BeverageSipper's Food Log

Breakfast   7:00 AM   **245 calories + 310 liquid calories**
2 cups bran cereal, ½ cup low-fat milk, 16 oz. orange juice, 1 cup coffee with vanilla-flavored Coffee-Mate (2 Tbs)

Snack   9:30 AM   **80 liquid calories**
1 cup of coffee with vanilla-flavored Coffee-Mate (2 Tbs), water

Lunch   12:00 PM   **280 calories + 220 liquid calories**
2 pieces whole grain bread, 4 Tbs. egg-white salad, 1 Tbs. lite mayo, celery & onion, 20 oz. bottle SoBe Green/Lemon Iced Tea

Snack   2:00 PM   **200 liquid calories**
Hot chocolate with whole milk

Dinner(out)   7:30 PM   **335 calories + 180 liquid calories**
Healthy Choice Lasagna Bake, side salad with lettuce, tomato, cucumber, and 1 Tbs light vinaigrette, 8 oz. glass red wine

Dessert   9:30 PM   **200 liquid calories**
Hot Toddy (2 oz. liquor)

Total Calories In = 1,970 + Liquid cals = 1,110!
Activities   1 hour walk (light)   **Total calories Out: 240**
Calories In – Calories Out = 1,730

Food Log Makeover

Nutrition Recommendations:

1. Don't drink so many calories. The RD gave BeverageSipper a calorie guide to make her aware of how the calories she drank were adding up. Hundreds of calories are in a single glass or bottle. By becoming aware of all calories, even liquids, Beverage Sipper would be better able to control her weight (and her blood sugar too). She was told to eat whole fruits instead of drinking juice. That way, she would consume fewer calories and more fiber. The RD also advised that BeverageSipper avoid calorie and fat-laden coffee creamers and substitute steamed skim milk. She was even told to watch alcohol, since those calories can really add up!

2. Drink more water. BeverageSipper was told to limit caffeine to about 200 mg/day and add 6 to 8 cups of water per day. The RD advised that she carry a water bottle with her at all times. In addition, BeverageSipper was told to drink decaffeinated beverages in order to stay hydrated. She was reminded not to underestimate fruits and vegetables, which are full of water too.

3. Keep daily food logs to monitor ALL calories. To get her on track, the RD had BeverageSipper make a beverage section on her daily log. At the end of the day, she had to tally up her food and liquid calories separately. This was to create initial awareness of her calorie intake.

4. Increase physical activity. Although she was off to a great start with light walking daily, if BeverageSipper increased to "moderate" walking, she'd burn an additional 3 calories/minute or 180 total calories. BeverageSipper's strength training was a great first step, and the RD encouraged her to talk with her trainer about increasing interval work.

Outcome:

Over the course of 4 months, Beverage Sipper became more aware of her total calorie intake. Keeping food logs really helped. Eventually, she wanted to save her calories for healthy foods and avoided liquid calories all together. BeverageSipper dropped ½ lb to 1 lb per week for a 12 lb weight loss. Her BMI dropped to 24 (within a healthy range) and her waist circumference decreased to 32 inches. As her fruit and vegetable intake increased, her cravings for sweets diminished and her hot flashes improved. Also, with her increased walking and strength training, BeverageSipper felt stronger every day. Even her blood sugar and cholesterol levels improved.

Food Log Makeover

Breakfast   8:00 AM   240 calories + 90 liquid calories

2 cups bran cereal, ½ cup skim milk, 1 orange, 1 cup of coffee with ½ c. steamed skim milk, water

Snack   10:30 AM   150 calories + 0 liquid calories

6 oz. container of low-fat cottage cheese, a small apple, water

Lunch   12:30 PM   280 calories + 2 liquid calories

2 pieces whole grain bread, 4 Tbs. egg-white salad, 1 Tbs. lite mayo, celery & onion, 20 oz. unsweetened decaf iced tea, water

Snack   3:00 PM   85 calories + 0 liquid calories

3:00 pm   1 small bag of baby carrots, 2 Tbs. hummus, water

Dinner   7:00 PM   335 calories + 90 liquid calories

Healthy Choice Lasagna Bake, ½ cup brown rice, Side salad with lettuce, tomato, cucumber, and 1 Tbs. light vinaigrette, 4 oz. glass red wine, water

Snack   9:00 PM   80 liquid calories

1 decaf Irish coffee, water

Total Calories In = 1,552 + 262 liquid calories = 1814 calories

Activity   1 hour "moderate" walk   = 420 calories burned

Total Calories In-Out = 1394 calories

Not All Carbs Are Created Equal

There are lots of healthy, high fiber carbs out there, like whole grains, beans, fruits, and vegetables. High-fiber carbs may help you eat fewer calories, and are ideal foods for people who are trying to control their weight and improve their health. Healthy high fiber carbs play a key role in many of the major food groups from MyPlate and are listed as helpful ways to get nutrients, according to the Dietary Guidelines for Americans.

Refined carbohydrate foods, on the other hand, do not necessarily have the same health benefits. In fact, some can be downright bad for you, especially when you eat a lot of them. Refined carbohydrate foods include things like cookies, crackers, cake, sugary foods, donuts, coffee cakes, muffins, waffles, pancakes, sweet cereals, packaged snack treats and chips, etc.

Glossary:

Refined carbohydrate foods: These are foods that have been processed from whole ingredients. Examples include sugar and flour, and foods made with these items as key ingredients. Refined foods usually lose fiber and important nutrients in the refining process. For example, white flour is a refined food made from whole wheat kernels. Sugar is a refined food made from sugar cane.

Refining foods increases their tastiness and calorie density. Delicious flavors and calorie density make it much easier to eat too many calories.

- Did you know that it takes 2,000 pounds of sugar cane to make 192 pounds of raw sugar? It is very easy to eat 100 calories worth of sugar, but very difficult to eat that amount from the sugar cane itself. (It's like eating bamboo).
- Compare grain products:
  - 8 ounces (1 cup) cooked whole wheat cereal: 149 calories
  - 8 ounces French bread: 403 calories
  - 8 ounces cookies: 1020 calories.

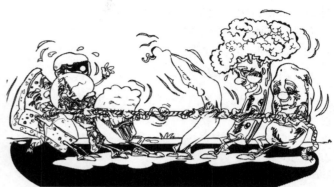

The more you refine foods (especially when adding sugars and fats) the more tasty and high in calories they become. Unfortunately for many, this process often makes the foods less healthy, yet more irresistable.

Whole plant foods: These are barely processed foods from plants that are in their whole, near-natural state. Whole plant foods are generally lower in calories, higher in fiber, and higher in nutrients than their refined counterparts. Examples of whole plant foods include fruits, vegetables, beans, and whole grains.

Whole foods are more filling and will make you feel more full on fewer calories.

- Compare potato foods:
  - 4 ounces baked potato = 82 calories
  - 4 ounces French fries = 348 calories
  - 4 ounces potato chips = 608 calories
- Fresh peaches contain 38 calories. The same amount of canned peaches in heavy syrup contains 73 calories - that's almost double!
- A 5-ounce apple has about 73 calories. A 5-ounce slice of apple pie packs 389 calories.

According to the National Weight Control Registry study, people who lost 30 or more pounds and kept it off for more than 1-2 years consumed a high-fiber, lowfat diet and exercised regularly. You can find out more about the study at *http://www.nwcr.ws/*.

Choose Preferred Carbohydrates

GO!—Preferred carbohydrates
Preferred high-carbohydrate foods are:

- Rich in water
- Rich in fiber
- Natural food – not concentrated, refined, or processed
- Low to moderate in calorie density

Nonstarchy vegetables are optimal foods for a weight-loss plan because their calorie density is so low. In fact, they only have around 65 to 195 calories per pound.

Fresh fruit is a delicious treat that is high in moisture and fiber. Whole fruit is preferable to dried fruit, fruit juice, or canned fruit in syrup. If you are purchasing canned fruit, try to find some that has been packed in water or its own juice.

Starchy vegetables and legumes are high in moisture and fiber, as well as being nutritious. Potatoes and sweet potatoes are easy to microwave and are great for lunch or snacks.

Cooked whole grains have high water content, are high in fiber, and fill you up with fewer calories than low-moisture items like bread or crackers. (White rice is lower in calorie density than white flour pasta). Cooked white rice and pasta are high in moisture, which means they are still low in calorie density and have around 517 calories per pound. If you don't like whole-grain items, these refined foods would be better than bread. Bread is more than double the calorie density of cooked rice, with 1224 calories per pound.

CAUTION: Cut Back on Calorie-Dense, Yet Nutritious, High-Carbohydrate Foods

While whole grain bread has 1224 calories per pound, it is not that much different (calorie-wise) from white bread, which has 1229 calories per pound. Whole grain bread is more nutritious than more processed bread, but it still should not make up the bulk of your diet, especially if you are trying to lose weight.

Dried fruit is another item that fits in the CAUTION category. It packs around 1360 calories per pound, so it should be eaten in moderation.

WHOA: Keep Intake of Refined, High-Carbohydrate Foods to a Minimum

What are refined carbohydrates?

- Refined starchy foods
- Foods high in refined sugars
- Foods with high calorie density
- Foods with little or no fiber

Examples of refined carbohydrates include: crackers, bakery items, donuts, bagels, cookies, pretzels, brownies, candy, bread, and cake.

Items made with white flour and sugar are very high in calorie density and usually contain little moisture or fiber. These foods should be a once-in-a-while treat rather than daily staples for people who want to lose weight.

The number of calories that you might find in a piece of cake is about the same as the number of calories in three baked potatoes. While it is much easier to eat a piece of cake than three potatoes, the three potatoes would make you feel fuller for longer. In fact, most people would have a hard time trying to eat three potatoes in one sitting.

Now, potatoes are not the same as cake, and cake can be a lot more delicious. This was simply an example to illustrate the idea that there's a wide gulf between GO and WHOA foods. If you're trying to lose weight, stick to the former.

Compare Carbohydrates

The calorie-light carbohydrate chart is very useful if you want to follow a diet that is low in calorie density, high in fiber, and full of nutrients. These items will help you feel fuller longer, with fewer calories too. They will also make you healthier by lowering your risk for many diseases... if you eat them on a regular basis. Eating the right carbohydrates is the key to a successful weight loss program.

The calorie-dense carbohydrate chart gives you an idea of foods that need to be limited and consumed infrequently for weight control.

Calorie-Light Carbs

Calories per pound:

Nonstarchy vegetables	65-195
Fruits	135-425
Skim milk	158
Hot cereal, unsweetened	242-281
Brown rice	488
Potatoes, yams	494
Barley	557
Whole-wheat spaghetti	562
Beans/legumes	576

These items contain fiber and moisture, but not any added fat or sugar.

Calorie-Dense Carbs

Calories per pound:

Bread	1,229	Baked potato chips	1,760
Ice cream	1,283	Doughnut	1,800
French fries	1,400	Croissant	1,800
Cake with frosting	1,544	Brownies	2,000
Unsweetened dry cereal	1,663	Snickers®	2,163
Pretzels	1,700	Cookies	2,200
Sweetened dry cereal	1,701	M&Ms®	2,272
Cheesecake	1,733	Potato chips	2,450

These items contain sugar and/or fat and have little fiber and moisture.

Advantage of Whole Plant Foods

Advantage of Whole Plant Foods

Take a look at the meals we profiled on this page. Note how the second section, which contains more natural and whole foods, weighs a lot more than the first section, even though both have roughly the same number of calories.

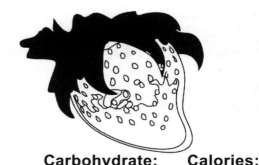

	Carbohydrate:	Calories:
Bagel Breakfast:		
1 bagel (4 ounces)	60 g	311
Light cream cheese	2 g	70
Milk, skim (1 cup)	12 g	85
Total	74 g	466
Total weight: 13 ounces		

	Carbohydrate:	Calories:
Oatmeal Breakfast:		
Cooked oatmeal (2 cups)	48 g	281
Skim milk (1 cup)	12 g	85
Orange (1)	15 g	61
Total	75 g	427
Total weight: 29 ounces	:	

• If you eat the Oatmeal Breakfast, you get twice the amount of food (by weight) than you would if you eat the Bagel Breakfast.

• The Oatmeal Breakfast contains 9 more grams of fiber and 10% fewer calories than the Bagel Breakfast.

• The Oatmeal Breakfast also contains 3 fewer grams of saturated fat and 751 fewer milligrams of sodium than the Bagel Breakfast, bringing it closer in line with MyPlate's recommendations.

	Carbohydrate:	Calories:
Macaroni & Cheese Dinner:		
Mac & Cheese (1 cup)	40 g	390
Salad (2 cups)	13 g	81
Apple sauce (1/2 cup)	22 g	86
Total	75 g	557
Total weight: 22 ounces		

	Carbohydrate:	Calories:
Stir-Fry & Brown Rice Dinner:		
Broccoli Stir-fry &		
Brown Rice (2 cups)	48 g	259
Salad (2 cups)	13 g	81
Diced Fruit (1 cup)	13 g	55
Total	74 g	395
Total weight: 27 ounces		

• You get 22% more food by weight when you choose the Stir-Fry over the Mac & Cheese, yet you'll keep the carb count just about equal to the other dish.

• The Stir-Fry has 162 fewer calories and 8 more grams of fiber than the Mac & Cheese.

• The Stir-Fry also contains 14 fewer grams of fat, 7.5 fewer grams of saturated fat, and 480 fewer milligrams of sodium.

Exercise more frequently and pinpoint the activities that you really enjoy. Those are the ones that will keep you coming back for more! Exercise often makes you crave the right carbs. Here are a few suggestions to help you switch from a refined-foods diet to a more whole-foods diet:

• Try baked potatoes instead of potato chips and french fries

• Eat salad or vegetable soup instead of deli sandwiches

• Start your day with cooked oatmeal instead of breakfast pastries

Delicious Recipes

Almond-Green Bean Salad

This delicious and crisp salad recipe is adapted from the Almond Board. You can find the original at *www.almondboard.com*.

4 cups butter lettuce, chopped

3 cups (~1 lb) frozen green beans, defrosted

1 cup cherry tomatoes, halved

1/3 cup sliced red onion

2 Tbsp balsamic vinegar

1 Tbsp olive oil

Black pepper to taste

2 Tbsp slivered almonds, toasted

Directions:

Rinse the lettuce in cold running water, drain it in the colander, then blot it dry with a paper towel. Mix the rest of the ingredients together in a large mixing bowl. Serve immediately or chill for up to 1 hour before serving.

Servings: Serves 4. Each 1.5 cup serving: 118 calories, 6 g fat, 0.6g saturated fat, 0 g trans fat, 0 mg cholesterol, 13 mg sodium, 14 g carbohydrates, 5 g fiber, 7.5 g sugars, 4 g protein.

Diabetic Exchanges:

Vegetable: 3.0

Total Preparation & Cooking Time: 10 min. (10 Prep, 0 Cook)

Arroz con Pollo

1 cup dry brown rice

2 cups water

3/4 cup roasted chicken breast, cubed

1/2 cup green peas

1/4 cup diced bell pepper

1/4 cup chopped green onion

1 teaspoon ground cumin

1 teaspoon coriander

1 teaspoon granulated garlic

1/4 teaspoon annato or paprika (for color)

Directions:

Place all ingredients into a rice cooker and cook until done, about 30 minutes. Serve hot.

This recipe goes well with a large tossed salad and is a great way to use up leftover chicken or turkey.

Servings: Serves 4. Each 1.5 cup serving: 244 calories, 1.4g fat, .4 g saturated fat, 0 g trans fat, 22 mg cholesterol, 23 mg sodium, 43.6 g carbohydrates, 2.5 g fiber, 1.9 g sugars, 12.7 g protein.

Diabetic Exchanges:

Bread & Starch: 1.5

Fat: 2.0

Lean Meat: 0.5

Vegetable: 1.0

Total Preparation & Cooking Time: 45 min. (15 Prep, 30 Cook)

Solve the Puzzle and Be Carb Smart

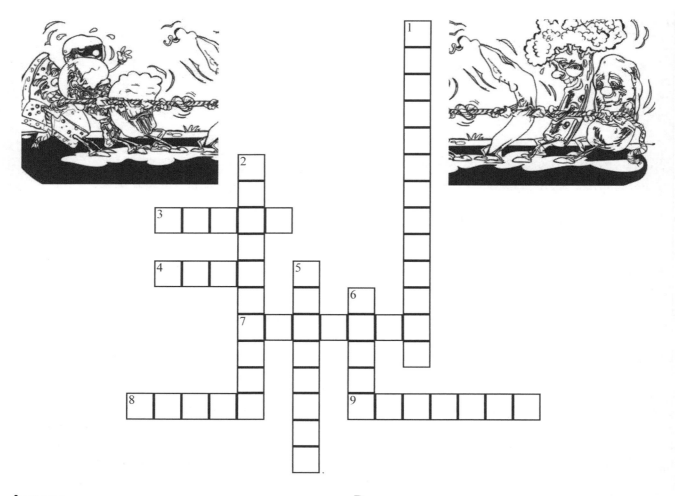

Across

3. Examples of this nutrient rich food group include bananas, oranges, and apples.

4. A cooked grain that is low in calorie density and eaten in great amounts in Asian cuisine.

7. A non-starchy vegetable used in salads.

8. An important part of plants that cannot be digested. Bran is one example.

9. Foods that have been highly processed from whole ingredients are said to be ___.

Down

1. The main energy source for the human body – one of the three main macronutrients. The other two are protein and fat.

2. A refined grain product that is in breads, crackers, and most baked goods; it contains the same amount of calories per pound as sugar.

5. A starchy vegetable that is fiber and nutrient rich. It is usually used baked or boiled.

6. A high-calorie, processed sweetener that adds calories, but no nutrients, to foods.

Answers:
Down: 1. carbohydrates, 2. whiteflour , 5. potatoes, 6. sugar
Across: 3. fruit, 4. rice, 7. lettuce 8. fiber, 9. refined

Out with the Bag!

Broccoli	9
Carrots	11
Apple	14
Yogurt, light	15
Pear	16
Banana	25
Baked potato	26
Muffin	80
Pretzel	82
French fries	87
Cinnamon Bun	96
Popcorn, light	101
Oreo	130
Chips	140
Chocolate Chip Cookie	141
Corn chips	150

Out with foods that are sold as snacks in all those cute packages and bags! Refined carbohydrates like muffins, pretzels, crackers, cookies, and chips are often high in sodium and fat and low in fiber. They are also often calorie dense and low in water content.

Take a look at the chart above. Compare the calories in the carrots, apples, and other items in the top half to the chips and cookies in the bottom half.

Just for laughs, here are the calories per ounce in common desserts. How do these compare to the chips and pretzels above?

Ice cream	**67**
Cheesecake	**89**
Brownie	**115**

When you're eating bagged snacks, it's hard to follow serving size recommendations. Luckily, there are now 100-calorie snack packs available in supermarkets. You can store a supply of these at home or in your locker to make sure you have an acceptable snack on hand. These packs are great for portion control, but are also expensive. You can make your own snack packs with Ziploc bags... just be sure not to leave large bags of food lying around! If you decide to go this route, divide the entire bag of snacks into single servings and put each serving in its own, smaller bag. Then it will be harder to snack mindlessly and pile on the calories. You could even make travel-ready baggies of fresh cut fruit or veggies for an ideal snack on the go!

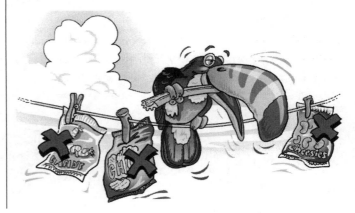

Successful Snacking Tips

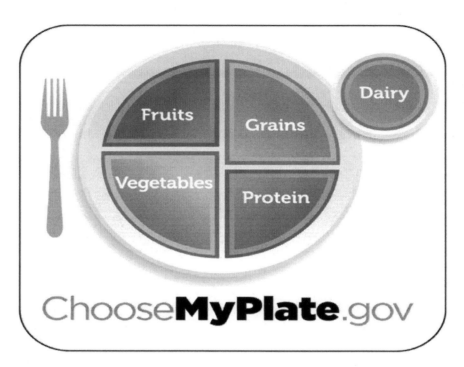

It's important to eat five to six smaller, more frequent meals instead on one or two larger meals, especially if you want to control your weight.

Healthful snacks act like bridges between meals and help you control your hunger. You should keep snacks to around 100-150 calories apiece. Remember to eat only when you are hungry, not out of boredom or anxiety. Healthy snacks are made from a variety of the foods recommended by MyPlate. Check out the food groups in the image above. What proportions are they in? What healthy foods fit in each group?

Keep an an abundance of the right foods on hand in your house. By controlling your environment (as much as you can) and having good choices available, you'll make it easier to make healthy decisions, even when you're in a rush.

For more information on MyPlate's food groups and healthful eating, visit *www,choosemyplate.gov*.

Stock up on nutritious foods:
- Oatmeal
- Air popped popcorn
- Whole grain crackers, bread, pitas
- Whole grain cereal
- Fresh vegetables
- Potatoes and sweet potatoes
- Fresh fruit
- Yogurt and skim milk
- Nuts
- Lean meat, poultry and fish

It's a good idea to write down what you eat along with the time and circumstances in which you eat it. That way, you will be able to identify eating patterns, danger situations, and whether you are going too long between meals. Remember, waiting until you are totally starving can set you up to overindulge later.

Super Snacks

Keeping the right foods on hand is very important for making fast, healthy snacks. If your snacks are based on whole grains, fruits, and vegetables, with a little fat-free dairy and lean protein, you will be on your way to better health. Here are some items you may want to have available:

Grains:
- Low-fat, whole-grain crackers
- Whole-wheat pita bread (100%)
- Whole-wheat bread (100%)
- Baked tortilla chips
- Whole grain cereal
- Air-popped popcorn

Vegetables:
- Raw vegetables
- Salads
- Potatoes and sweet potatoes
- Vegetable juice (100%)
- Vegetable soups

Fruits:
- Fresh fruit
- Dried fruit

Heart Healthy Protein:
- Nuts and nut butters
- Bean dip
- Bean soup
- Bean salad
- Canned tuna or salmon
- White meat from chicken or turkey, skinless

Heart Healthy Dairy:
- Nonfat, light yogurt
- Skim milk

Easy Snack Ideas
For healthy snacks, get rid of refined carbohydrates like pretzels, crackers, cookies, and chips. These snacks are often high in sodium and fat, while staying low in fiber. They are also calorie dense, which makes it easy to eat too many calories without thinkings. Here are some healthy snack ideas:

- **Peanut butter crackers** - This old standby is a great choice when made with 100% whole grain, lowfat crackers. Keep the peanut butter to 1 tablespoon and top with fresh sliced fruit.
- **Soup** - Purchase low-sodium, low-fat vegetable or bean soup. It can be microwaved in minutes in a coffee mug.
- **Rabbit bag** - Put a few raw veggies and fruits together in a zip lock bag. Use orange wedges, apple slices, raw cauliflower, and raw carrots. The orange gives everything a nice flavor and will keep the apple slices from discoloring.
- **Smoothie** - Blend skim milk and fruit to make a delicious drink that tastes like a milk shake.
- **Low-sodium vegetable juice** is a great way to increase your consumption of veggies in a pinch.
- **Tuna on toast** - Make a tuna salad with low-fat mayonnaise. Spread it on a slice of toasted 100% whole wheat bread and top with sliced tomato and lettuce.
- **Oatmeal raisin bowl** - Make a bowl of oatmeal with raisins and cinnamon, top with skim milk.
- **Cereal parfait** - Layer light, nonfat yogurt, fruit, and whole-grain cereal in a cup
- **Baked sweet potato** - "Bake" it in the microwave and top with reduced calorie pancake syrup and a pinch of cinnamon.

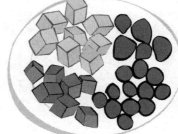

Snack Recipes

Strawberry Sparklers

Serve these strawberries for a healthy snack or delicious dessert.

1 lb fresh, large strawberries

1 cup light cream cheese

1/2 cup diced or chopped almonds

2 Tbsp rainbow sprinkles

Directions:

Wash strawberries under cold running water to remove any excess dirt. Pat them very dry with paper towels. Place cream cheese in a small glass bowl, cover and microwave until soft and warm, about 30-45 seconds. Stir well. Place chopped almonds and colored sprinkles in a small bowl. Dip strawberries in cream cheese then in nut/sprinkle mixture. Place them on a small plate. Once the plate is filled with strawberries, stick it in the refrigerator to firm up the cream cheese. Serve chilled. You will have 1/2 cup of cream cheese left over; reserve it for another use.

Servings: Serves 6. Each serving (4 ounces): 131 calories, 9 g fat, 3 g saturated fat, 0 g trans fat, 2 mg cholesterol, 202 mg sodium, 3 g carbohydrates, 2 g fiber, 12 g sugars, 4 g protein.

Diabetic Exchanges:

Fruit: 0.5

Milk: 1.0

Total Preparation & Cooking Time: 10 min. (10 Prep, 0 Cook)

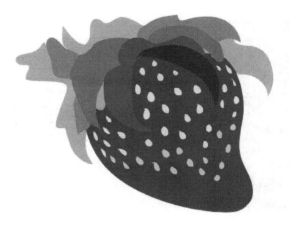

Parsley Hummus

1 15-oz can garbanzo beans, rinsed and drained

1/4 cup water

1 tablespoon olive oil

2 tablespoons lemon juice

2 cloves garlic, minced

1/2 cup chopped parsley

Directions:

In a food processor or blender, combine all ingredients except parsley and process until smooth. Add the parsley and pulse or stir to incorporate. Serve as a spread or dip alongside bread, crackers, or fresh vegetables.

Servings: Serves 8. Each serving: 1/4 cup: 71 calories, 2 g fat, 0 g saturated fat, 0 g trans fat, 0 mg cholesterol, 137 mg sodium, 11 g carbohydrates, 2 g fiber, 0.1 g sugars, 2.5 g protein.

Diabetic Exchanges:

Bread & Starch: 0.5

Total Preparation & Cooking Time: 5 min. (5 Prep, 0 Cook)

Snack Recipes

Maple Baked Sweet Potato

1 sweet potato

1 teaspoon light margarine

1 tablespoon low-calorie maple syrup

Directions:

Wash the sweet potato under cold running water and pierce the skin several times with a fork. Put it in the microwave and cook on full power until tender, about 5-6 minutes. Turn once halfway through cooking. When the potato is done, cut it in half and top with light margarine and low-calorie syrup.

Servings: Serves 1. Each serving: 1 potato: 188 calories, 1.5 g fat, 1 g saturated fat, 0 g trans fat, 0 mg cholesterol, 71 mg sodium, 41 g carbohydrates, 4.5 g fiber, 0 g sugars, 2 g protein.

Diabetic Exchanges:

Bread & Starch: 2.0

Vegetable: 1.0

Total Preparation & Cooking Time: 10 min. (5 Prep, 5 Cook)

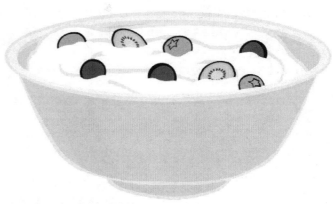

Vanilla Fruit Parfait

2 cups cubed peaches

1 cup sliced strawberries

1 cup lowfat vanilla yogurt

1 firm, medium banana, peeled and sliced

1/3 cup raisins

1/4 cup sliced almonds, toasted

Directions:

Layer peaches, strawberries, yogurt, banana, and raisins equally in four glasses and sprinkle the tops of each with almonds.

Servings: Serves 4. Each serving: 1 cup: 181 calories, 4 g fat, 0.6 g saturated fat, 0 g trans fat, 4 mg cholesterol, 46 mg sodium, 48 g carbohydrate, 4 g fiber, 38 g sugars, 4.5 g protein.

Diabetic Exchanges:

Bread & Starch: 3.0

Fruit: 2.0

Total Preparation & Cooking Time: 15 min. (15 Prep, 0 Cook)

Case Study: Consistent Meal Skipper

Skipping meals throughout the day causes overeating, slowed metabolism, and weight gain.

Meet Meal Skipper:

Height	5'10"
Weight	220
BMI	35
BMI category	Obese Class II
Waist Circumference	44"

Notes:

MealSkipper presented to a registered dietitian (RD), complaining of fatigue and lack of energy. His medical history revealed Class II obesity, high cholesterol, high blood pressure, and slightly impaired glucose tolerance (pre-diabetes). MealSkipper's life has became sedentary and he spends a great deal of time sitting at the office. In fact the only activity he gets comes in the form of daily walks to the train station (~ 2 blocks). He says his wife is a great cook and often makes elaborate dinners.

Upon nutrition assessment, MealSkipper was able to discuss a typical day in no time flat, since he claimed "not to eat a lot." He was baffled by his weight gain over the years because he didn't eat much during the day. He only eats breakfast on the weekends (and he treats it more like brunch), lunch consists of a quick sandwich or soup, chips, and a diet soda. Although he doesn't characterize himself as someone who adores chocolate, MealSkipper does have a 3:00 pm snack of a handful of the M&Ms on his secretary's desk. By dinner, he is extremely hungry. From the moment he walks in the door at 6:00 pm, the first thing he does is open the refrigerator and wait for something to pop out at him. He typically reaches for a slice or two of cheese and salami.

Dinner usually consists of meat, potatoes or rice, and vegetables with "some sort of sauce." He always has seconds.

Nutrition Assessment:

Upon looking at the composition of MealSkipper's diet, his thought process seemed to indicate that if he skipped breakfast he would be saving calories for later. However, he makes up for the missed calories (and more!) during the day. By not eating anything until 12:30 pm – MealSkipper guarantees that he is quite hungry and will eat more than he would if he had eaten breakfast. Moreover, both his calorie and fat intake were over and above healthy limits. MealSkpper cannot afford to eat over 2,000 calories in a day because he doesn't exercise.

MealSkipper was honestly unaware of his calorie intake and thought it was much lower. With the help of the dietitian, he created a plan to change his lifestyle during the next month.

A Day in the Life of MealSkipper

Breakfast   6:00 AM   0 calories

Large glass of water

Lunch   12: 30 PM   770 calories

Au bon pain vegetarian chili in a bread bowl, diet soda

Snacks   430 calories

3:00 PM   ¼ cup plain M&M candies

6:00 PM   2 slices mozzarella cheese, 2 slices of hard salami, 1 beer

Dinner (home)   7:00 PM   965 calories

2 slices of Meatloaf (6 oz.) , ¾ c. mashed potatoes w/ pat of butter, 1 c. broccoli w/ 1 oz. cheddar cheese sauce, water

Snack   10:00 PM   260 calories

1 cup vanilla ice cream, water

Total Calories In = 2,633

Walk – 1/4 mile to/from train, 100 calories burned

2,633 – 100 = 2,533 Calories for the day

Food Log Makeover

Nutrition Recommendations:

1. Do not skip meals or snacks. The RD gave MealSkipper a list of healthy, high fiber breakfast options and informed him that he needs to get approximately 30 grams of fiber per day. Breakfast is the perfect time to eat whole grains. By filling up on fiber in the morning, MealSkipper is less likely to overeat at his other meals. He was also told to set calorie limits for 2,000 calories per day. Breakfast = 350, Lunch = 650, Dinner = 700 + 2 snacks = 150 calories per day (300 calories). He should eat less food, more frequently and was told not to go longer than 5 hours without a meal or snack.

2. Eat less saturated fat. MealSkipper needs to watch for hidden saturated fats in deli meats, cheese, sauces, and full-fat desserts. The RD recommended that he keep fat to around 30% of his total calories, with two thirds of that amount coming from "good" fats, like olive oil, canola oil, almonds, and walnuts.

3. Keep daily food logs with calorie counts. MealSkipper was shocked to see the number of calories he ate in one day. When what you eat is logged daily, it increases awareness of several things including portion sizes, quality, timing of meals, and hunger cues.

4. Drink more fluids. Do not underestimate the fact that water fills you up, yet has zero calories. MyPlate advises people to replace sugary drinks with water.

5. Increase physical activity. The RD advised MealSkipper to aim for at least 30-60 minutes of activity on most days of the week. According to the Dietary Guidelines for Americans, in order to stave off chronic disease, adults should engage in at least 30 minutes of moderate-intensity physical activity, above and beyond their usual activity, on most days.

Outcome:

MealSkipper almost reached his goal of 10% weight loss within 6 months of working with the RD. He was down ~7 % of his body weight. His Body Mass Index dropped to 33 and he lost 2 inches in his waist. He also increased his activity to the recommended 30 minutes per day. MealSkipper spread his meals out throughout the day and did not skip any meals or healthy snacks. His breakfast was always high fiber and low-fat. Throughout the day, MealSkipper monitored the amount of fat and sodium he ate. He did not feel the need to go back for second helpings at dinner. Soon, he went to bed less full and slept better through the night.

Food Log Makeover

Breakfast   7:00 AM   355

1 Natural Ovens whole grain bagel, 1 tablespoon natural almond butter, 1 medium orange, 8 oz. water

Snack   9:30 am   130

1 small banana, 3 sesame rye crackers, water

Lunch   12:30 PM   615

15 oz. Health Valley vegetarian chili, 1 slice Natural Ovens bread, 1 small salad (lettuce, tomato, cucumber) with 2 tablespoons balsamic vinaigrette, 1 medium apple,

Snack   3:30 pm   155

String cheese, ½ cup baby carrots + 2 tablespoons hummus, water

Dinner   7:00 pm   470

4 oz. turkey meatloaf (93% lean), 1 medium baked potato, 1 tablespoon fat-free sour cream, 1 cup of broccoli sprinkled with 1 tablespoon grated Parmesan cheese, water

Snack   9:00 pm   90

1 cup green tea, 2 whole grain Fig Newtons

Total Calories In = 1,815 (~ 718 calories deficit = - 1 ½ lb/week)

What Is Fat?

Fat is one of the three macronutrients that supply calories to the body. The other two macronutrients are carbohydrates and protein. Fat has nine calories per gram. Carbohydrates and proteins have only four calories per gram.

Different Types of Fat

Saturated fat is solid at room temperature. Unsaturated fat is liquid at room temperature.

Foods that are high in *cholesterol* also tend to raise blood cholesterol. These foods include liver and other organ meats, egg yolks, and dairy fats.

Trans fat is found in fat that was liquid at room temperature but was made solid by a process called hydrogenization. You usually see this in fried foods or food that includes partially hydrogenized shortening.

Unsaturated fats (oils) do not raise blood cholesterol. Unsaturated fats can be found in vegetable oils, most nuts, olives, avocados, and fatty fish like salmon. Unsaturated oils include both monounsaturated fats and polyunsaturated fats. Olive, canola, sunflower, and peanut oils are all high in monounsaturated fats. Vegetable oils like soybean oil, corn oil, and cottonseed oil, as well as many kinds of nuts, are all good sources of polyunsaturated fats. Some fish, (such as salmon, tuna, and mackerel) contain omega-3 fatty acids that are seem to offer protection against heart disease. Eat a small amoutn of food that is high in unsaturated fats.

Fat's Duties

- Energy source
- Insulation for the the body
- Storage for fat calories
- Aid for transport and absorption of fat-soluble vitamins
- Sustainer of healthy skin and hair

Notes About Fat from the Dietary Guidelines for Americans

- Get less than 10 percent of your total daily calories from saturated fatty acids. Eat less than 300 mg/day of cholesterol. Avoid trans fatty acids whenever you can.
- Keep fat to between 20 to 35 percent of your total calories. Have most fats coming from sources of polyunsaturated and monounsaturated fatty acids, like fish, nuts, and vegetable oils.
- When choosing and cooking meat, poultry, dry beans, and milk (or milk products), make choices that are lean, low-fat, or fat-free.
- Limit the amount of fats and oils high in saturated and/or trans fatty acids that you eat. Choose products low in these fats and oils.

Essential fatty acids must come from dietary fat – your body can't make them itself. It is important to eat a healthy diet in order to get the right nutrients, and some of these nutrients include essential fatty acids. Do not lower the fat in your diet to less than 8-10% of the calories you consume daily, though it is wise to keep the total percentage of fat in your diet to less than 30%.

How Much Fat Do You Need?

Dietary fat provides essential omega-3 and omega-6 fatty acids. In a 2,000 calorie diet, the average person would need about:

- 1-2 g of omega-3
- 4-8 g of omega-6

These amounts can be found easily in 8-10% of the calories from fat in a healthful diet.

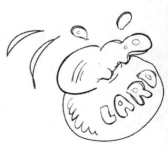

Fat is Calorie Dense

Low Calorie Density

The items on the following chart are all relatively low in calorie density and high in moisture and fiber. They are also low in fat. Listing foods by calories per pound is a good way to compare their calorie densities.

Category Density	Products	Calories per pound	Calorie
Vegetables	all	65-195	very low
Fruits	all except avocado	135-425	low
Nonfat dairy	nonfat milk, yogurt	180-400	low
Egg whites	nonfat egg substitute	226	low
High-water carbs	potato, peas, beans, pasta, rice, barley, cooked cereals	300-600	moderately low
Poultry & fish	lean poultry lean fish, shellfish	450-650	moderately low

High Calorie Density

Fat is an energy-dense food, in a much higher calorie range than fruits, vegetables, and the other foods shown in the chart above. It is important to choose your fats wisely. Nuts, avocadoes, and olives all have good fats. Cheese, fatty meats, fried foods, and processed foods have fats that are harmful for your heart. Remember, if you lower the fat in your diet, you should not replace it with refined carbohydrates like sugar.

Category Density	Products	Calories per pound	Calorie
Cheese, egg yolks	cheddar, Swiss, Brie	1,500-2,000	high
Processed foods	potato chips, cookies, salad dressing, candies, brownies, fudge, crackers	1,500-2,500	very high
High-fat products	chocolate candy, peanut butter, nuts, seeds	2,500-3,000	very high
High-fat products	bacon, butter, mayo	3,000-3,500	very high
Fats, oils	olive oil, vegetable oil, shortening, lard	4,000	extremely high

Where is the Fat?

Where Is the Fat?
- Fatty meats
- Dairy products:
  - Butter
  - Whole milk
  - Cheese
- Refined fats and oils:
  - Salad dressings, oils, margarine
  - Fried foods, many restaurant foods
  - Most desserts
  - Many frozen dinners
  - Processed foods
- Nuts and nut butters

A quick note about nuts and nut butters: These foods are nutrient-dense and contain important minerals. They can be part of a weight loss plan but should be included rarely.

Managing Fat in the Kitchen
- Use **skim milk** in place of whole milk: You will save 5 grams of saturated fat per cup by using skim milk or calcium-fortified soy milk instead of whole milk

- Use **light margarines** for spreads. The best versions contain less than 1 gram of saturated fat and 50 calories or fewer per serving.

- Use **less refined oil**:

  – In most cases you can cut the amount of oil recommended in a recipe by half.

  – Measure oil, don't pour it freely.

  – Use a spray can or misting bottle for distributing oils.

  – Use broth for flavoring and sauteeing. It's especially great for finishing vegetables or pasta.

- Choose **lean cuts of meat and trim all excess fat**. White skinless poultry is lower in fat than many cuts of red meat. Lean ground turkey is also low in fat, and is often best used in recipes with a little liquid. If ground turkey contains dark meat and/or skin, it can often be as high in fat and saturated fat as ground beef.

- **Choose lowfat cooking methods** like baking, grilling, roasting, poaching, microwaving, and steaming.

- Instead of a whole egg, **use two egg whites** or ¼ cup nonfat egg substitute.

- **Cheese** is very high in fat and saturated fat. Try extra sharp cheddar or Parmesan, which both have a lot of flavor and can be used in small doses.

- Use **fat-free salad dressing** or a small amount of oil and vinegar to dress salads. Or dip your fork in the dressing, then grab a bite of veggies, rather than the other way around.

- When dining out, **order sauces on the side**. Choose lowfat items and smaller portions. In some restaurants, you can even ask them to use lowfat cooking methods.

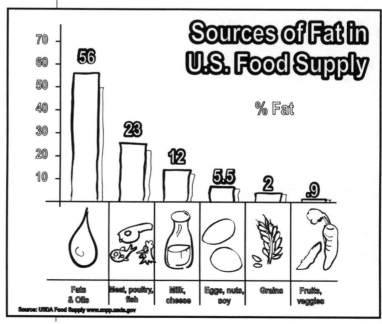

Sources of Fat in U.S. Food Supply

% Fat

Source: USDA Food Supply www.cnpp.usda.gov

Lowfat Recipes

Baked Parmesan Chicken

Bread crumbs and Parmesan cheese give chicken a crispy, savory coating. This recipe saves 155 calories and 11 grams of fat per serving compared to a fried chicken breast.

4 boneless skinless chicken breast halves

1 cup nonfat plain yogurt

3/4 cup plain bread crumbs

4 Tbsp. Parmesan cheese

2 Tbsp. all-purpose flour

1 tsp. paprika

Pinch of cayenne pepper

Directions:

Place chicken breast halves in yogurt and refrigerate while you prepare the rest of the food. Mix the remaining ingredients in a medium-sized mixing bowl. Preheat oven to 425° and lightly spray a cookie tray with vegetable cooking oil.

Coat each piece of chicken with yogurt and dredge through the crumb mixture, pressing down on both sides and turning over several times to get a thick coat of crumbs. Place chicken on the tray and spray the top with vegetable cooking oil. Bake breasts for 15-20 minutes or until chicken is fork tender and its juices run clear.

Servings: Serves 4. Each serving: ½ breast: 280 calories, 6 g fat, 2 g saturated fat, 0 g trans fat, 75 mg cholesterol, 420 mg sodium, 22 g carbohydrates, 1 g fiber, 4 g sugars, 34 g protein.

Diabetic Exchanges:

Bread & Starch: 1.5

Lean Meat: 3.0

Total Preparation & Cooking Time: 35 min. (15 Prep, 20 Cook)

Spinach Salad

This delicious salad is high in flavor and low in fat!

1 cup nonfat vanilla yogurt

2 Tbsp red wine vinegar

1 Tbsp honey

1 tsp prepared mustard

6 cups fresh spinach, washed and ready to serve

1/4 cup sliced red onion

1/2 sliced apple

1 orange, peeled and diced

Directions:

Combine the first 4 ingredients in a large mixing bowl. Add the rest of the ingredients, toss, and serve. You can also chill the salad for up to one hour before serving.

Servings: Serves 4. Each serving: 1 cup: 79 calories, 0.3 g fat, 0 g saturated fat, 0 g trans fat, 1 mg cholesterol, 108 mg sodium, 16.1 g carbohydrates, 5.8 g dietary fiber, 12.6 g sugars, 3.9 g protein.

Diabetic Exchanges:

Bread & Starch: 1.0

Vegetable: 3.0

Total Preparation & Cooking Time: 5 min. (5 Prep, 0 Cook)

Sample Lowfat Meal Plan

Breakfast:

Oatmeal with skim milk

1 banana

½ cup berries

Coffee or tea

Cooked oatmeal or cream of wheat is an excellent choice for breakfast because its calorie density is much lower than the calorie density of bagels, danish, croissants, and even dry processed cereals. Compare this breakfast with a McDonald's Sausage Biscuit with egg (which has 490 calories and tons of sodium, not to mention its fat content and lack of fiber).

Lunch:

Large salad with 1 tsp oil & vinegar

Large bowl of chicken minestrone soup

1 slice of 100% whole-grain bread

Diet soda or tea

This lunch is very generous. You get to eat a large, four-cup salad with oil and vinegar (use 1 tsp of oil and as much vinegar as you like) plus a two-cup bowl of minestrone soup and a slice of 100% whole wheat toast. Enjoy unsweetened tea or water along with your meal.

Snack:

Yogurt with fresh fruit and whipped cream

Herb tea

This snack combines one cup of light, nonfat, flavored yogurt with a half cup of fruit and one tablespoon of fat-free whipped cream. Enjoy flavored herb tea on the side.

Dinner:

Baked lemon fish

Red-grilled potatoes

Sautéed spinach

Fresh tomatoes

Enjoy four ounces of your favorite fish baked with herbs, fresh lemon, and paprika. Bake it in a dish with a little water to make sure that it stays moist. Add two cups of baby spinach. Grill red potatoes with a little olive oil, onion, and tomato paste and top with chopped tomato. Remember to drink water with dinner.

Dessert: Banana Sundae

Dessert isn't just for little kids. Make a delicious banana sundae with nonfat, light vanilla yogurt, a half slice of banana, a half cup of fresh berries, sprinkles, 1/2 tablespoon of chocolate chips, and reduced-calorie chocolate syrup. Top with one tablespoon of fat-free whipped cream.

Meal Plan Stats

1,700 calories

31 g fat

6 g saturated fat

100 mg cholesterol

2,572 mg sodium

282 g carbohydrate

42 g fiber

87 g protein

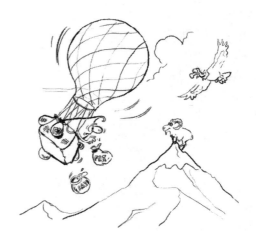

Case Study: FatSlurper

Eating high fat, high calorie foods throughout the day packs on pounds.

Meet FatSlurper

Female, late 20s

Height	5'4"
Weight	198
BMI	34, (Class I)
Waist Circumference	37"

Notes:

FatSlurper went to a registered dietitian (RD) complaining of recent weight gain, especially "around the middle." Her medical history revealed Class I obesity, borderline high blood pressure, elevated fasting blood sugar, and recently diagnosed polycystic ovarian syndrome (PCOS). FatSlurper was interested in starting a family soon, so her doctor recommended that she see an RD, especially because nutrition plays a big role in fertility. In fact, it plays a particularly large role in dealing with PCOS.

Upon nutrition assessment, FatSlurper mentioned that she used to like vegetables and fruit, but has not had a taste for them in a while. Over the last year (after her wedding) she and her husband have been too busy to cook and have fallen into the habit of dining out often. FatSlurper was quick to qualify where they ate as "not fast food places or anything like that." According to FatSlurper, she was not a snacker and only ate an occasional cookie in the afternoon. Her typical dinner always included high fat, fried foods. She and her husband would usually order fatty appetizers or add on an order of fries to share. With no motivation to work out, FatSlurper was depressed about her weight, but felt helpless to control it.

When the RD calculated the amount of fat that FatSlurper's ate, she discovered that it was almost 40% of her total calories. FatSlurper wasn't aware of all the hidden fats in her meals and snacks, and her fiber intake was really low. With no physical activity, her weight just kept climbing.

Nutrition Assessment:

FatSlurper was clearly overeating, in terms of both fat and calories. By not eating vegetables and fruit, her diet had almost no fiber and antioxidants. She dined out for practically every meal. If she was going to continue eating out, FatSlurper had to changeher food choices. She also needed to learn how to snack in a healthy manner.

FatSlurper's lack of activity was not helping her body burn many of the calories that she ate. In fact, as her body fat increased, her muscle mass decreased. In effect, her body fat (biologically inactive tissue) was greater than her muscle mass (biologically active tissue).

A Day in the Life of FatSlurper

Breakfast   8:00 AM   585 cal/26 g fat

4 ounce muffin, 1 grande latte (whole milk)

Lunch   12: 30 PM   1270 cal/52 g fat

1 cup Sticky Thai Rice (with coconut & sesame seeds), 1 chicken satay, diet soda

Snack   3:00 PM   280 cal/13 g fat

1 large Mrs. Field's chocolate chip cookie + 1 cup water

Dinner   7:30 PM   940 cal/40 g fat

1 hamburger with cheese, 1 small order of French fries, 1 chocolate milkshake

Total Calories In = 3,075 (38% from fat)

Activity Calories Out: None

Food Log Makeover

Nutrition Recommendations:

1. Eat smart when dining out. FatSlurper needs to focus on getting more vegetables, high fiber carbs, and lean protein (like chicken, fish, and tofu) when dining out. The RD also gave her a dining out guide, which focused on how to cut fat from her meals.

2. Eat healthy snacks. The RD told FatSlurper to eat at least 2-3 snacks per day and to aim for snacks with high dietary fiber and low fat content. The RD even gave FatSlurper a list of healthy snacks. In accordance with the Dietary Guidelines for Americans, FatSlurper's goal became getting at least three 1-oz. servings of whole grains a day. The RD informed her that her fiber needs are about 25-30 grams/day. FatSlurper needs to eat less, more often and not go longer than 4-5 hours without a meal.

3. Eat less fat, especially saturated fat. FatSlurper was told to ask that food be prepared with cooking spray instead of oil or butter. She also needs to watch for hidden saturated fats in deli meats, cheese, sauces, and full-fat desserts. FatSlurper should keep fat to ~ 25-30% of the total calories she consumes (50 g in an 1,800 calorie diet). She also has to aim for getting 10% or less from saturated fats and 20% from "good" fats, like olive oil, canola oil, almonds, and walnuts. The RD reminded her that even good fat has calories, so she should measure ALL fats.

4. Keep daily food logs with calorie, fats and fiber grams. The idea here is to eat mindfully. The premise of the mindfulness-based eating approach (see the Center for Mindful Eating's website at *www.tcme.org*) is that chewing slowly, savoring every bite, and being aware of what you are eating helps stave off overeating and helps you make healthy choices.

When you log your food intake daily, it can increase your awareness of portion sizes, quality of food intake, timing of meals/snacks, and hunger/fullness cues. That's why FatSlurper needs to start a food log.

5. Increase physical activity. The RD informed FatSlurper about the Borg Scale for rating physical activity. She was advised to strive to go from 6 (which is no physical activity) to at least a 13 (somewhat hard). She had to start with about 30 minutes of activity (i.e., walking) most days per week, and lift weights too

Outcome:

FatSlurper cut her fat intake significantly over the course of 9 months. She was aware of what she was ordering at restaurants, making desserts and appetizers the exception, rather than the norm. She lost 12% of her body weight. FatSlurper also started walking to and from work (about 2 miles each way) and lifting light weights when she got home from work. Her family even started cooking at home about 3 nights per week.

Food Log Makeover

Breakfast   8:00 AM   285 cal/6 g fat

1 ½ c. Fiber One cereal, ½ cup skim milk, 1 small apple, 1 grande soymilk latte

Snack   10:30 AM   140 cal/1.5 g fat

6 oz. Stonyfield lowfat vanilla yogurt, water

Lunch   12:30 PM   445 cal/6.5 g fat

Subway 6" Oven Roasted Chicken Breast sandwich, 1 bag baked chips, water

Snack   3:00 PM   170 cal/15 g fat

1 oz. almonds, 8 oz water

Dinner   7:00 PM   640 cal/9.5 g fat

1 cup minestrone soup, salmon over a bed of greens, ½ cup brown curry rice, water

Snack   9:00 PM   120 cal/2.5 g fat

½ cup low-fat ice cream, 1 cup green tea

Total Calories In = 2070

(41 grams/fat = 18% fat)

Cooking is the Better Weigh

"There are a number of reasons for people to increase the percentage of meals and snacks they prepare themselves. Among these is the need to

1. increase the amount of fiber- and nutrient-rich ingredients,
2. control the type and quantity of fat used,
3. limit the amount of added sugar and salt, and
4. adjust portion size to actual caloric need."

— Melanie Polk, RD, American Institute for Cancer Research (*www.aicr.org*)

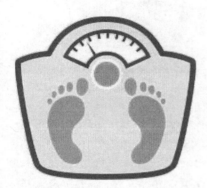

Cooking at home saves time. After all, it takes almost 80 minutes to eat at a restaurant (if you consider the time you leave your driveway until the time you get home). A survey of food and nutrition professionals indicated that almost 75% could put dinner on the table in 30 minutes or less. With a little bit of creativity and know-how, you can too!

Eating at home costs a lot less. You don't have to pay someone else to prepare your food, let alone worry about tips and service charges. The chart at right demonstrates how you can save a bundle on dinner for four by cooking at home.

When you're trying to lose weight, perhaps the most important savings of all comes in terms of calories. The chart at the top of this page shows the difference between restaurant items and the same foods cooked at home. You can control the amount of fat and sodium that goes into your food, as well as portion size, when you cook a meal in your own kitchen.

Save Calories:

Restaurant		Home-Cooked
773	Lemon Pepper Fish	346
766	Grilled Chicken	434
700	Gourmet Pizza Slice	308
650	Lasagna	340
644	Pasta Pomodoro	302
624	Clam Chowder	210

Save Time:

Eating out:
Driving – 20 minutes
Dining – 60 minutes
= 1 hour, 20 minutes

Cooking at home:
Prep time – 30 minues
Dining – 15 minues
= 45 minutes to cook and eat

The times for this comparison come from the average times given in an extensive survey performed by Food and Health Communications.

Save Money:

Homemade spaghetti and salad for 4:

Jar of sauce:	$3.19
Box of spaghetti:	$1.00
Romaine:	$1.19
Tomatoes:	$2.10
Cucumber:	$1.40
Total:	**$8.88**
Minutes to prepare:	**15**

4 spaghetti and salad dinners at a restaurant:

Per person*:	$10.99
Total:	**$43.96**
Minutes to pick up:	**30-45**

Not including beverages, tax and tip

How to Cook a Better Weigh

You can cook healthy meals at home without sacrificing flavor. It's easy to make your own recipes a little lower in fat and calories – you just need a little know-how and the right ingredients. Check out some of our fat zapping tips below.

Cook With Little Fat

The way you prepare food can affect its fat content just as much as the ingredients you use. For example, a healthy meal can become a calorie bomb when fried. Try these tricks to keep the fat content under control.

- Nonstick skillets usually need very little fat for cooking, since you don't have to create a stick resistant layer with oil or butter.
- To keep fat low, bake, broil, microwave, grill, or steam your food.
- Avoid frying and pan frying. Most recipes can be baked instead. You can also use less oil/fat when you do decide to fry.
- De-fat gravy with a special cup (called a fat separator). You can also chill gravy, which causes the fat to rise and harden at the top. Chip off the fat and reheat the rest before serving.

Reduce the Fat: Refined Oil

Use fat-free salad dressing or a small amount of oil and vinegar instead of heavier dressings.

If you carefully measure the oil you use, you'll wind up using much less than you would if you poured the oil freely.

Choose Lean Protein

- Chicken or turkey: white meat, no skin
- Tenderloin of beef or pork loin
- Seafood (without breading or heavy sauce)
- Trim excess fat before cooking.
- Remember, a 3-ounce serving of meat is the size of a deck of cards.

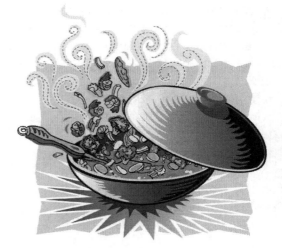

Choose Fat-Free Dairy

According to MyPlate, people should choose low fat and nonfat versions of dairy foods whenever possible. There are lots of products on the market to help you make better choices in the dairy case. Consider these:

- Skim milk
- Fat-free sour cream or Greek yogurt
- Light margarine (look for trans fat free)
- Fat-free half-n-half
- Reduced fat cheese

Use More Fruits and Vegetables

Most fruits and vegetables are naturally low in fat and sodium. Plus, they pack quite a nutritional punch. Add more vegetables to casseroles, soups, stews, and pasta dishes.

For More Information

www.foodandhealth.com
www.choosemyplate.gov
www.cookinglight.com
www.foodfit.com
www.americanheart.org

Stock Your Kitchen for Fast Meals

The secret to preparing fast and delicious meals at home is to have the right ingredients on hand. Make sure you or your parents have picked up the pantry staples listed below. Having these items available will enable you to cook quick and healthy meals at any time of day.

To get the most out of your time in the kitchen, follow the advice of over 400 food and nutrition professionals and make planned leftovers! When you cook, make extra servings to freeze or serve the next day.

Dry Goods for the Pantry

Canned or dry beans

Lentils

Your favorite spices, herbs, and seasonings

Healthful canned soups

Oil and vinegar

Pasta

Pasta sauce

Rice

Tuna fish

Whole-grain breads and cereals

Staples in the Refrigerator

Fruits

Vegetables

Salad fixings

Potatoes

Sweet potatoes

Fat-free sour cream

Margarine (light)

Orange juice

Parmesan cheese

Skim milk

Yogurt (light)

10 Fast Meal Ideas:

1. Baked potato stuffed with fat-free sour cream, steamed broccoli, and Parmesan cheese; tossed salad

2. Baked chicken or fish; steamed rice; salad or fresh vegetables

3. Spaghetti with lentils and pasta sauce; salad

4. Macaroni with turkey tomato sauce; salad

5. Shrimp vegetable stir fry with rice

6. Chili (vegetarian or with ground turkey breast); brown rice; salad

7. Veggie burger with a baked sweet potato; fresh-steamed vegetables

8. Tuna macaroni casserole (add tuna and vegetables to box mix, omit margarine, and only use half of the powdered sauce packet).

9. Vegetable soup

10. Chicken stew

Recipes available at *www.foodandhealth.com*

Food for the Freezer

Chicken

Ground turkey breast (skinless)

Fish and seafood

Lean cuts of beef or pork (loin or round)

Frozen, chopped fruit

Frozen, chopped vegetables

Nuts

Veggie burgers

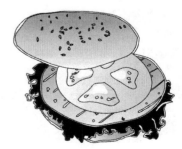

Recipe Modification

Instead of:	Portion	Saturated fat (g)	Use:	Saturated fat (g)
Dairy:				
Butter	1 Tbsp	7.5	Vegetable oil* or broth	0
Cream	2 Tbsp	7	Evaporated skim milk	0
Cream cheese	2 Tbsp	6.5	Light cream cheese	3.5
Half and half	2 Tbsp	2	Fat-free half and half	0
Hard cheese**	1 ounce	6	Low-fat cheese+	1
Ice cream	1/2 cup	6	Frozen yogurt	1.5
Ricotta cheese	1/2 cup	10	Fat-free ricotta	0
Sour cream	2 Tbsp	3	Fat-free sour cream	0
Whipped cream	2 Tbsp	3	Fat-free whipped cream	0
Whole milk	1 cup	5	Skim milk	0
Whole milk	1 cup	<u>5</u>	1% milk	<u>1.5</u>
Totals		**61**		**7.5**

*Use a spray oil or cut amount in half.

**Cut amount of cheese in half or use a small amount of Parmesan cheese

+Add on top at end of baking for best results

Meat/Poultry				
Bacon	3 slices	3	Turkey bacon	1.5
Beef, ground	3 ounces	7	Ground turkey breast, no skin	0
Beef, ground	3 ounces	7	Vegetarian burger*	0
Beef, prime rib**	3 ounces	12	Beef tenderloin, fat trimmed	3
Beef, T-bone	3 ounces	7	Beef tenderloin, fat trimmed	3
Chicken, dark with skin	3 ounces	3	Chicken breast, no skin, baked	.5
Chicken, fried thigh	1 each	6	Chicken breast, no skin, baked	.5
Lard	1 Tbsp	5	Margarine, trans-fat free	2
Sausage	3 ounces	<u>9</u>	Vegetarian sausage*	<u>0.5</u>
Totals		**54**		**11**

*Read the label, nutrition facts vary by brand

**Restaurant portions are often triple this amount.

Note: For heart-healthier cooking, limit animal protein and emphasize whole grains, beans, soy protein, fish, fruits, and grains in your meals; think of meat as a side dish and use less of it.
A 3-ounce serving of meat is generally the size of a deck of cards.

Miscellaneous				
Coconut milk	8 ounces	20	Evaporated skim milk	0
Whole eggs	2	3	Egg white or nonfat egg substitute	0
Gravy with fat	2 Tbsp	5	Defatted gravy	0.5
French fries	4 ounces	4	Baked potato	0

How to Get Organized in the Kitchen

Do you want to lose weight? Are you ready to try cooking for yourself or your family? Do you want to make and eat healthy and delicious meals?

If you answered yes to any of these questions, then keep reading! (If not, you should keep reading anyway. Maybe we'll change your mind). We are going to explore ways to eat more healthfully while spending less time and money on food and and food prep.

Cooking can be fun, but it's also a bit hard, especially if you've never done it before. With just a little know how, however, you can prepare simple, healthy meals for less than most people spend on groceries.

One great strategy is to cook large batches of food and freeze the extras in small, portion-sized packages. To make "planned overs" a breeze, all you need to do is follow these five steps...

1. Clean and organize your freezer. Your parents will thank you. Just be sure you check with them before throwing things away. Remember, you'll need space for anything you want to freeze.

2. Purchase clear, freezable, microwaveable containers or bags. These will store your food, so be sure to have them readily accessible. On the shelves in the grocery store is not accessible enough when you have the remains of a pan of lasagna to freeze.

3. Make large batches of your favorite recipes freeze the rest in individual portions. Be sure to label the things you freeze with their contents and the day they were made. Try freezing cooked beans, cooked rice, cooked pasta, lasagna, spaghetti, pasta, soups, rice, healthful macaroni and cheese, and stir-fry dishes. Not all foods will freeze successfully, so you may want to experiment.

You don't have to have a cooking marathon and make a ton of food in one day, and you don't have to cook food solely to freeze it. Simply cook in order to prepare a meal, then freeze the extras.

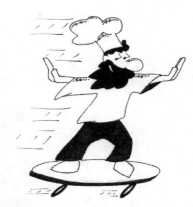

Making a double batch is helpful, but not required.

4) Cool foods down quickly. Soups, beans, and other large dishes should be cooled in a shallow container in the refrigerator so you don't increase your risk of getting food poisoning.

5) Reheat items quickly in the microwave. Usually you just need to add a little water and cover whatever you're heating with a lid or plastic wrap. Items in plastic bags should be moved to a microwaveable container before reheating.

If you are preparing items that are based on beans and whole grains, they will cost less than entrées that center around meat. Eating at home rather than eating out will save your family both time and money. You will save time because you won't be traveling to a restaurant and spending time waiting to be seated, served, and presented with a check. You'll save money because you won't have to pay food preparation costs, or tip any waiters. Food that is prepared at home is often lower in sodium and fat than restaurant meals or frozen prepared items from grocery stores.

For more information about food safety, visit: *http://www.fsis.usda.gov/Fact_Sheets/Cooking_for _Groups_index/.*

Fast and Easy Meals

Mexican Lasagna

16 oz fat-free ricotta cheese
16 oz reduced-fat ricotta cheese
 1 tsp garlic powder
 1 tsp dried oregano leaves
16 corn tortillas
52 oz low-sodium pasta sauce (2 jars)
 1 cup shredded light mozzarella cheese

Preheat oven to 350 °F. Mix ricotta and seasonings in bowl. Layer lasagna in a 9"-by-12" pan. Layer sauce, tortillas, ricotta filling, and repeat in that order as necessary. Top with more sauce, then sprinkle with mozzarella cheese. Cover with foil and bake for one hour or until heated through. Allow lasagna to stand for 5 minutes, then cut into 10 cubes and serve hot.

Nutrition Facts: Serves 10. Each serving: 354 calories, 9 g fat, 4 g saturated fat, 22 mg cholesterol, 392 mg sodium, 47 g carbohydrate, 6 g fiber, 19 g protein.

Turkey Chili

2 tsp vegetable oil
1 onion, chopped
 1/2 lb lean, skinless, ground turkey breast
15 oz (1 can) pinto or kidney beans, with juice
15 oz (1 can) diced tomatoes, no added salt
 1/2 tsp garlic powder
 1/2 tsp chili powder
 1/3 cup water

 Heat the vegetable oil in a Dutch oven or large pan over medium-high heat. Sauté the onion briefly and add the ground turkey. Cook until the turkey is no longer pink, then add the rest of the ingredients. Bring to a boil. Lower heat and simmer for 10 minutes.

Nutrition Facts: Serves 4. Each serving (1 cup): 181 calories, 3 g fat, 0.5 g saturated fat, 22 mg cholesterol, 373 mg sodium, 20 g carbohydrate, 7.5 g fiber, 18 g protein.

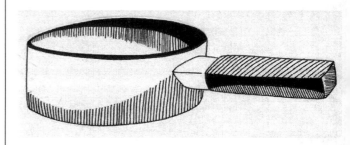

Roasted Tomato Spaghetti

12 oz boxed spaghetti
4 ripe tomatoes, cored and halved
 1/2 onion, cut into chunks
1 green pepper, cut into chunks
1 Tbsp olive oil
2 Tbsp chopped fresh basil
1 tsp garlic powder
Black pepper (to taste)

 Cook spaghetti according to package directions. Drain and reserve in colander. Meanwhile, make the sauce. Preheat oven broiler. Place vegetables on a cookie sheet and broil for 20 minutes until golden. Flip vegetables halfway through cooking. Place the vegetables, olive oil and seasonings in a food processor or blender and blend on high speed until smooth. Heat sauce and serve over pasta. Top with Parmesan cheese.

Nutrition Facts:

Serves 4. Each serving: 383 calories, 5 g fat, <1 g saturated fat, 0 mg cholesterol, 13 mg sodium, 72 g carbohydrate, 4.5 g fiber, 12 g protein.

Fast and Easy Meals

Arroz con Pollo Express

1 cup cooked chicken breast cubes, without skin
1 tsp ground coriander
1 tsp ground cumin
1 cup frozen peas and carrots
1 cup long-grain brown rice
2 cups chicken broth

Rice cooker directions: Place all ingredients in rice cooker and cook until done, about 30 minutes.

Stove-top directions: Place all ingredients in large pan. Bring to a boil over medium-high heat. Lower heat to simmer. Cover pot and cook over low heat until rice is done, about 30 minutes.

Serve hot alongside a large salad.

Nutrition Facts: Serves 4. Each serving: 270 calories, 3.5 g fat, 0.5 g saturated fat, 42 mg cholesterol, 181 mg sodium, 39 g carbohydrate, 3 g fiber, 19 g protein.

Chili Rice Pot

1 cup instant brown rice
15 oz canned diced no-salt-added tomatoes with juice
15 oz canned pinto beans, drained and rinsed
1/2 cup water
1 tsp chili powder

Place all ingredients into a 2-quart microwaveable container. Cover and microwave on high until rice is done, about 8-10 minutes. Stir well and serve hot.

Nutrition Facts: Serves 4. Each serving: 181 calories, 1 g fat, 0 g saturated fat, 0 mg cholesterol, 237 mg sodium, 37 g carbohydrate, 7 g fiber, 7.5 g protein.

Spaghetti with Lentils

1 cup dry lentils
8 oz package dry spaghetti
26 oz jar pasta sauce, preferably low sodium
1 tsp Italian seasoning
4 Tbsp Parmesan cheese

Directions:

1. Place a large soup pan filled with water over high heat and bring to a boil. Add the lentils and return to a boil.

2. Lower heat to medium and cook for 4 minutes then add spaghetti. Bring water back to a boil over high heat and cook until spaghetti is al dente and lentils are tender, about 10 minutes. Drain in colander.

3. Place the same pot back on the stove and add the pasta sauce and Italian seasoning. Bring to a boil, then add the pasta and lentils. Heat through and serve immediately.

Serves 4. Each 1 and 1/4 cup serving: 382 calories, 2.5 g fat, 1 g saturated fat, 4 mg cholesterol, 680 mg sodium, 72 g carbohydrate, 6 g fiber, 17 g protein.

Fast Meal Assembly

Are you one of the many people that do not like to cook or follow recipes? The good news is that there are a lot of fast and easy dishes that you can "assemble" without following an exact recipe. Here are a few of our favorites:

Baked potato and salad

Baking potatoes

Nonfat sour cream

Prepackaged lettuce

Seasonal vegetables

Flavored vinegar

Seasonings

Directions: Bake potatoes in microwave. Prepare salad in a large bowl and serve with vinegar. Serve the potatoes with the nonfat sour cream and seasonings.

Pita pizza and salad

Whole wheat pita pockets

No-added-salt pasta sauce

Veggies

Grated Parmesan (use rarely)

Prepackaged lettuce

Seasonal vegetables

Flavored vinegar

Directions: Preheat oven to 350. Top pitas with pasta sauce and veggies and bake until cheese melts, about 12 minutes. Prepare salad in a large bowl and serve with flavored vinegar.

Pasta and salad

Your favorite pasta

No-added-salt pasta sauce

Grated Parmesan (use rarely)

Prepackaged lettuce

Seasonal vegetables

Flavored vinegar

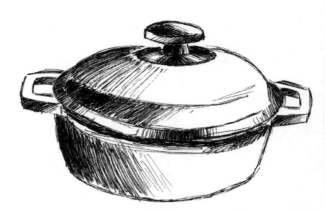

Make pasta according to package directions. Heat sauce and mix with pasta. Prepare salad in a large bowl and serve with flavored vinegar.

Microwave fish meal

Fresh or thawed fish filets (not breaded)

Lemon

Powdered garlic and parsley mix

Baking potatoes

Steamed veggies

Nonfat sourcream

Place fish filets on a microwave-safe platter with a little water and cover. Microwave on fish setting or until done, about 2 minutes per filet. Microwave potato and veggies. Serve potatoes with nonfat sour cream. Serve fish and veggies with lemon and a sprinkle of garlic/parsley seasoning.

Chicken Stir Fry

Steamed rice

Chunks of chicken breast

Frozen stir fry vegetables

Light soy sauce and sesame oil

Steam rice according to package directions. Cook chicken and vegetables in a wok with just a little oil. Cook until chicken is completely done and veggies are tender. Season them with light soy sauce and sesame oil.

Fast Food Facts

Since the 1970s, the amount of fast food that Americans eat has dramatically increased. About 50% of the money people spend on food is spent on food that is eaten in restaurants. Just to compare, in 1955, only 25% of food money was spent in restaurants. French fries, hamburgers, and pizza are the most popular items consumed. Did you know that over 500 billion will be spent this year on meals outside of the home? After all, fast foods are generally appealing and portion sizes are large.

Why be concerned about fast foods?

1. **Obesity** is skyrocketing in the United States, in both adults and children. There is more Type II Diabetes today than at any other time in history. Other health concerns associated with high body weight include heart disease, certain cancers, and high blood pressure. Most fast food choices are calorie dense and nutrient poor, which makes them bad choices for fighting obesity and managing weight.

2. **Soda has replaced milk** at most fast food restaurants. A child-sized soda usually contains 12 ounces of liquid and has 150 calories. Medium and large sodas have between 200 and 300 calories.

3. **Artery-clogging fat:** Fast foods are high in fats, especially saturated fat and trans fat. High fat diets have been linked to heart disease, cancer, and many other health problems.

4. **Missing fiber and nutrients**: Whole grains, fruits and vegetables... where are they? You won't find many whole grain, fruit, or vegetable choices in the majority of fast food restaurants.

5. **Children**: Today, kids are getting an average of 10% of their daily energy from fast foods. Children are encouraged to eat fast food through TV commercials, toys, restaurant playgrounds, and other marketing strategies.

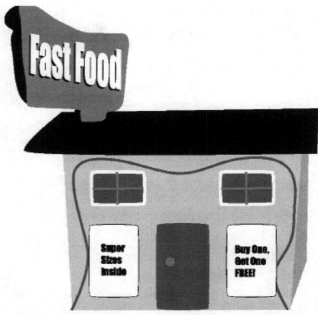

In the past 20 years, kids have experienced great increases in body fat. Larger calorie intake, as well as decreased activity, are two possible explanations for this dramatic increase. In fact, children are now expected to die at a younger age than their parents.

So why do we choose fast foods?

- **Simplicity**: Purchasing foods that are already prepared takes less time, eliminates clean up, and is often less expensive than cooking at home. You can pick up on the way home from school or as part of a sit-down meal at your favorite restaurant.

- **Variety**: There are many fast food restaurants to choose from. Since 20 years ago, the number of different restaurants and chains has increased 4 times over.

- **Super size**: Fast food restaurants offer large portions for a low price. That means that we feel like we are receiving a lot of food, especially given the money we spent.

Fast Food: Whoa! Know Before You Go!

Fast food is here to stay. The guidelines below will help you make better choices to eat healthier and avoid weight gain.

- **Plan ahead**. Most fast food restaurants have websites that list nutrition information for all their food. Plan your meals to be around 400 calories, with less than 15 grams of fat.

- **Avoid extra calories**. Ask for the dressings, sauces, sour cream, and butter that go with your dish to be served on the side. Skip cheese and fried items.

- **Say no to super sizes and large portions**. The larger portion may only be a few cents more, but MyPlate advises people to avoid oversized portions.

- **Don't eat in the car**. Bring your food home or eat it in the restaurant. When people grab good "on the run" they are less aware of how much they actually eat.

- **Choose foods that are grilled, baked, or sautéed**.

- **Load sandwiches with as many vegetables** as you can add.

- Chicken items are not always that low in fat or sodium - sometimes a **plain hamburger** is a better option.

- Try a **meatless meal** for a change: Burger King has a veggie burger and Subway has a vegetable sandwich. Cheese or veggie pizzas are available at most pizza chains too. However, most of these choices are not low in sodium.

- **Choose reduced calorie dressings** or bring your own. You can get the same flavor for half of the calories. Choosing a fat free dressing will further reduce calories.

- **Order whole grain breads** when possible. Whole grains fill you up faster and contain fiber and other nutrients that are simply not available in white bread.

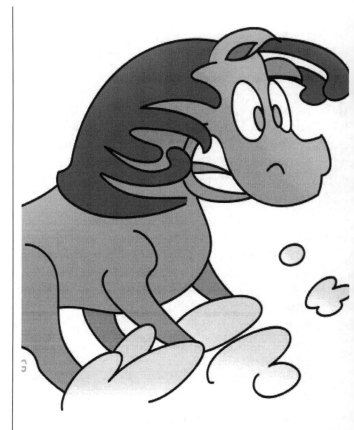

Ethnic Choices:

- **Mexican restaurants**: Order flour tortillas instead of hard shell tacos or larger burritos. Limit the amount of cheese and choose items that are not deep-fried.

- **Chinese restaurants**: Order meat items that also include with vegetables. Stay away from deep fried egg rolls, wonton skins, and fried rice. Share your entree with someone else order a meatless entree. Serve it over steamed rice.

- **Italian restaurants**: Marinara sauce has a lot less fat and calories than alfredo sauce. Limit the amount of garlic bread and spaghetti you eat. Order items with only a little meat and cheese. Limit pizza to one slice and have a big salad along with it.

Hunt for Fast Food Facts

www.bk.com – For Burger King's nutrition information, go to the menu and click on its links.

www.chipotle.com - The homepage has a quick link for nutrition information near the top left of the menu.

www.dominos.com – Their nutrition information is broken down into four categories – a calorie counter, ingredient information, allergen information, and a list of light options.

www.fastfood.com/nutrition/ – This one-stop site lists nutrition information for numerous fast-food restaurants.

www.hardees.com – When you look at the online menu, you can access nutrition information with one additional click.

Nutrition Facts for Your McMeal

Bag a McMeal

[Recalculate] [Add Item] [More Details]

		Calories	Total Fat (g)	Saturated Fat (g)	Cholesterol (mg)	Sodium (mg)	Carbohydrates (g)	Dietary Fiber (g)	Protein (g)
☑	Grilled Chicken Bacon Ranch Salad	250	10	4.5	85	930	9	3	31
☑	Crispy Chicken Bacon Ranch Salad	370	21	7	65	1040	20	3	26
☑	Grilled Chicken Caesar Salad	200	6	3	70	820	9	3	29
☑	Crispy Chicken Caesar Salad	310	16	4.5	50	890	20	3	23
☑	Grilled Chicken California Cobb Salad	270	11	5	145	1060	9	3	33
☑	Crispy Chicken California Cobb Salad	380	23	7	125	1170	20	3	27
	Total:	*1770*	*87*	*31*	*545*	*5910*	*88*	*18*	*168*
	% Daily Value**:	-	133	154	182	246	29	70	-

www.kfc.com – Take a look at their online nutrition guides and ingredient statements.

www.mcdonalds.com – You won't just find nutrition info on this site. Keep your eyes peeled for discussions of their ingredients and a guide to children's nutrition too.

www.panerabread.com - You may be surprised about just how many calories their simple sandwiches, salads, and baked goods contain.

www.pizzahut.com – The nutrition information is a bit hard to find here, but it is, in fact, available. Look to the little links at the very bottom of the page.

www.starbucks.com – In addition to a long list of nutrition info, this site also includes lists of drinks with less than 200 calories, and foods with 10 g of fat or fewer.

www.subway.com – Look at the top of the home page for nutritional information.

www.tacobell.com – Their nutrition section also includes a calorie calculator.

www.wendys.com – It's hard to see all the nutrition info at once here. Instead, there is a menu you use to select nutrition info for a category of food, like burgers or shakes. Then you can look for individual items from there.

Keep Fast Food Heart Healty

Here is a cheat sheet of fast food items that don't go over 600 mg of sodium per serving and have reasonable amounts of calories, fat, and saturated fat. Think of these as a last resort in a pinch.

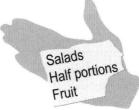

Salads
Half portions
Fruit

	CALORIES	FAT (g)	SATURATED FAT (g)	SODIUM (mg)
BURGER KING				
Whopper Jr or Burger (no cheese/mayo)	260	10	4	460
Garden Salad	70	3.5	2	90
Fresh Apple Fries	70	0.5	0	40
McDONALD'S				
Small Hamburger	250	9	3.5	520
Side Salad (no dressing)	20	0	0	10
Oatmeal w/ Cranberries, Raisins, Apples	260	4.5	2	115
Apple Dippers with Caramel Dip	100	0.5	0	35
Low-fat Ice Cream Cone	150	3.5	2	60
Snack Sized Fruit & Walnut Salad	210	8	1.5	60
PANERA BREADS				
½ Kids Peanut Butter/Jelly	205	9	1.75	275
½ Asian Sesame Chicken Salad	205	10	1.75	405
5 oz. Fresh Fruit Cup	60	0	0	15
PIZZA HUT				
*Fit Chicken, Onion, Green Pepper	180	4.5	1.5	510
*Fit Ham, Pineapple, Tomato	160	4.5	1.5	550
*Fit Green Pepper, Onion, Tomato	150	4	1.5	400
SUBWAY				
6" Veggie Delite	230	2.5	0.5	310
Grilled Chicken and Baby Spinach Salad	130	2.5	0.5	330
Veggie Delite Salad (no dressing)	50	1.0	0	65
TACO BELL				
Fresco Grilled Steak Soft Taco	150	4	1.5	520
Fresco Grilled Chicken Soft Taco	150	3.5	1	480
WENDY'S				
Junior Hamburger	250	10	4	640
Garden Side Salad	210	13	2	400
Baked Potato, plain	270	0	0	25
Apple Slices	40	0	0	0

List compiled by Sarah Mohrman, RD, MA, Fort Wayne Cardiology.

Low-Cal Fast Food Choices

Restaurant	Food Item	Calories	Fat Grams
Burger King	Whopper Junior	340	19
Burger King	Veggie Burger	410	16
Burger King	Hamburger	260	10
Chick Fil-A	Chargrilled Chicken Cool Wrap	410	12
Chick Fil-A	Chargrilled Chicken and Fruit Salad	220	6
Culver's	Original Butter Burger Single	331	16
Culver's	Garden Fresco Salad (no dressing)	229	10
Culver's	Grilled Chicken Sandwich	310	4
Dairy Queen	Original Cheeseburger	400	18
Dairy Queen	Grilled Chicken Sandwich	370	16
Domino's Pizza	12 inch - Hand Tossed Onions and Peppers	185	6.5
Domino's Pizza	12 inch - Hand Tossed Pacific Veggie	230	10
Domino's Pizza	12 inch - Deep Dish Pepper and Onion	230	9.5
Fazoli's	Spaghetti and Marinara (kids size)	220	1
Fazoli's	Meat Lasagna (kids size)	260	13
Fazoli's	Fettucine Alfredo (kids size)	290	8
Hardee's	Trim-It Charbroiled BBQ Chicken	170	3.5
Hardee's	Grits	110	5
McDonald's	Snack Sized Fruit Walnut Salad	210	8
McDonald's	Asian Grilled Chicken Salad	270	9
McDonald's	Plain Hamburger	250	9
Panera Bread	Garden Vegetable Soup with Pesto	150	5
Pizza Hut	12 inch - Chicken, Onion Peppers	180	5
Pizza Hut	12 inch - Ham, Pineapple, Tomato	160	4
Pizza Hut	14 inch - Hand Tossed Veggie Lover's	290	9
Subway	6 inch - Turkey Breast	280	3.5
Subway	6 inch - Veggie Delight	230	2.5
Taco Bell	Two Fresco Chicken Soft Tacos	300	7
Taco Bell	Fresco Burrito Supreme - Chicken	350	8
Taco Bell	Fresco Bean Burrito	350	8
Wendy's	1/2 Apple Pecan Chicken Salad (no dressing)	280	15
Wendy's	Ultimate Chicken Grill Sandwich	390	10
Wendy's	Baked Potato with Sour Cream and Chives	320	4

Beware of High Calorie Fast Food

Restaurant	Food Item	Calories	Fat Grams
Burger King	Whopper with Cheese	710	43
Burger King	Triple Whopper with Cheese	1,180	78
Burger King	Double Croissant (egg, cheese, sausage)	700	49
Chick Fil-A	Spicy Chicken Sandwich Deluxe	570	27
Chick Fil-A	Chicken, Egg, and Cheese Bagel	490	20
Culver's	Butterburger Double Deluxe	712	47
Culver's	Cheddar Butterburger with Bacon, Double	761	49
Culver's	Shaved Prime Rib Sandwich	507	29
Dairy Queen	1/2 lb Flame Thrower Burger	1010	71
Dairy Queen	Chicken Strip Basket (4pc with gravy)	1160	47
Fazoli's	Twice Baked Lasagna	700	39
Fazoli's	Submarino Sandwich - Original	880	49
Fazoli's	Tortellini and Sun-Dried Tomato Rustico	850	46
Hardee's	Thickburger	850	57
Hardee's	Loaded Breakfast Burrito	760	49
Hardee's	1/3 lb Original Thickburger	770	48
McDonald's	Big Breakfast with Hotcakes and Large Biscuit	1150	60
McDonald's	Chicken Selects Breast Strips (5)	640	38
McDonald's	Cinnamon Melts	460	19
Panera Bread	Frontega Chicken Panini	850	38
Panera Bread	Sierra Turkey	920	49
Panera Bread	Italian Combo Sandwich	980	41
Pizza Hut	14 inch Meat Lover's Pan Pizza	480	28
Subway	Chicken and Bacon Ranch	570	28
Subway	Meatball Marinara	560	24
Taco Bell	XXL Grilled Stuft Burrito - Chicken	840	35
Taco Bell	Fiesta Taco Salad	770	42
Taco Bell	XXL Grilled Stuft Burrito - Beef	880	42
Wendy's	Bacon Deluxe Single Burger	670	40
Wendy's	BLT Cobb Salad	650	46
Wendy's	Bacon and Cheese Baked Potato	520	20

4 Easy Ways to Make Better Fast Food Choices

At some time during a typical week, a person is likely to be hungry when a healthy, prepared meal is unavailable. If that person is currently driving (alone or with friends/family), s/he might be tempted to stop at a fast food restaurant. In fact, this happens to a lot of people. Sales for quick-service restaurant operators are supposed to increase to $137.8 billion, according to the National Restaurant Association's publication, *Restaurant Industry Forecast – 2003*.

This page will help you make a better choice the next time you enter a fast food restaurant. Here are some facts to consider from Marylou Anderson, RD, a nutritionist at a community health center in Seattle:

- A supersized soft drink (42 oz) has 136 grams of sugar. That's 34 teaspoons of sugar!

- A Kentucky Fried Chicken Oven Roasted Strips Meal (3 Oven Roasted Strips, Green Beans, Seasoned Rice) has 2410 milligrams of sodium, which is a whole day's supply for most people.

- A Burger King Fish Fillet Sandwich and medium serving of French fries has 5-1/2 tablespoons of fat (61 grams).

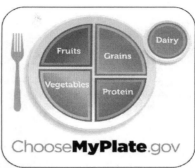

Marylou offers 4 easy ways to lower the amount of fat, sodium and calories that you consume in a fast food meal:

1. Choose baked, grilled, or broiled items instead of fried foods. Salads, grilled chicken, baked potatoes, and small lowfat sandwiches are always your best choices.

2. Put condiments on the side and only use them occasionally.

3. Order unsweetened tea, or water instead of soda or other sweetened beverages.

4. Don't super size your meals. Fast food nutrition information can be found at the restaurants' websites. Most have calculators to help you make a better decision by adding up the toal calories in your meal.

Fast Food Quiz

It pays to know before you go. Sometimes a food that sounds healthy is not really a great choice when it comes to calories. Here is a quiz to put you in the know. Choose the lowest calorie item for each set below:

1. A Taco Bell Fiesta Taco Salad or a McDonalds Big Mac

2. Super sized French fries or a Quarter Pounder with Cheese

3. An Egg McMuffin or a Sausage Biscuit with Egg

4. Wendy's Junior Bacon Cheeseburger Classic Single a Wendy's Bacon and Cheese Potato

Answers:

1. A Fiesta Taco Salad from Taco Bell has 770 cals), while a Big Mac has 540 cals.

2. A super sized order of fries has 540 calories. A Quarter Pounder with Cheese has 510.

3. An Egg McMuffin has 300 cals, while a Sausage Biscuit with Egg has 510 cals.

4. Wendy's Junior Bacon Cheeseburger Classic Single w/ everything has 400 calories, and a Wendy's Bacon and Cheese Potato has 520. Betcha didn't see that one coming, did you?

Fast Food Trivia

Super Sized Portions	Calories:
Whopper with cheese, mayo	850
Large fries	500
Large soda	330
TOTAL	**1,680**

Regular Portions	Calories:
Hamburger, no mayo	280
Salad with fat-free dressing	135
Diet soda	0
TOTAL	**415**

The next time you order out, consider that super sizes may pose a danger to your health and waistline.

Here are some fun trivia questions to help you do better when you eat at the drive-thru.

1) How many calories are in a 42 ounce soda?
a) 350 calories
b) 420 calories
c) 525 calories

2) A 42 ounce soda would contain how many cans of soda?
a) 1.5 cans
b) 2.5 cans
c) 3.5 cans

3) How many grams of trans fat are in large fries?
a) 2 g
b) 3 g
c) 7 g

4) How many calories do you save by ordering a hamburger with no mayo versus a large whopper with cheese and mayo?
a) 300 calories
b) 570 calories
c) 600 calories

5) French fries made in oil without trans fat have how much trans fat?
a) 0 g
b) .5 g
c) 7g

6) Trans fats:
a) raise LDL, aka "bad cholesterol"
b) lower HDL, aka "good cholesterol"
c) both a and b

7) What are better options than fried food?
a) fruit
b) salad
c) all of the above

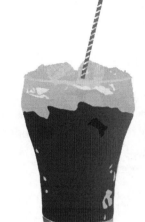

Answers:
1) c) 525
2) c) 3.5
3) c) 7
4) b) 570
5) b) 0.5
6) c)
7) c)

Don't Let the Salad Fool You!

Just because a menu item is a salad doesn't mean that it's low in calories. In fact, some salads can pack a bigger wallop than a small burger or even fries! Know before you go!

Salad	Source	Calories	Fat(g)
Chick-N-Strips Salad with Ranch Dressing	Chick-Fil-A	620	39
Chicken Cashew Salad with French Dressing	Culvers	663	36
Pasta Ranch Italia Salad	Fazoli's	770	50
Fuji Apple Chicken Salad	Panera	560	34
Steak and Blue Cheese Chopped Salad	Panera	860	61
Fiesta Taco Salad	Taco Bell	770	42
Baja Salad	Wendy's	730	47
BLT Cobb Salad	Wendy's	650	46

The Healthy Plate

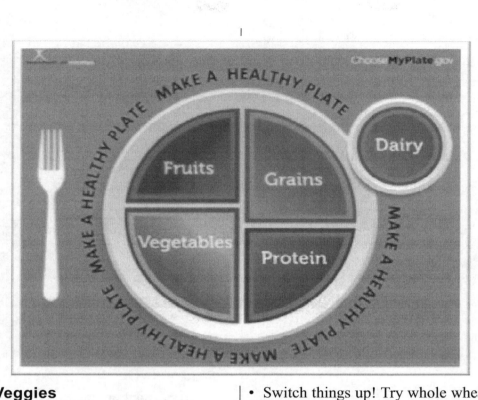

Fruits and Veggies

- Most people need 4.5 cups of fruits and vegetables per day (that's about 1.5 cups per meal). For a personalized recommendation, visit *choosemyplate.gov*.
- Eat a variety of colors of fruits and veggies: dark green, orange, blue/purple, white, or red.
- *MyPlate recommends that you fill half your plate with fruits and vegetables at each meal.*

Lean Protein

- Most people need between 5 and 6 ounces per day.
- Be sure to include seafood and beans each week.
- Choose protein items that are lean and prepare them in a healthy way (poaching, grilling, etc).
- *MyPlate advises that people chooose a variety of lean protein sources.*

Whole Grains

- Most people need to eat around 6 ounces of grains per day.

- Switch things up! Try whole wheat pasta, brown rice, oats, barley, millet, and quinoa.
- *MyPlate recommends that people make half the grains they consume whole grains.*

Dairy

- Most people need around 3 cups of dairy per day.
- Steer clear of saturated fat, sodium, and added sugar by checking the Nutrition Information.
- *MyPlate advises that people stick to to lowfat or nonfat versions of milk, yogurt, and cheese.*

Downsize your plates!

Consider downsizing your dishes, bowls, and cups. Smaller plates will help you serve less food without feeling deprived. After all, smaller bowls and plates look more full with less food on them than larger bowls and plates do.

Try using the dinner plate for a large, lowfat salad and then use the salad plate for your dinner.

Visit *foodandhealth.com/blog* for more tips, tricks, recipes, and photos.

Compare Plates

The diagram below shows that the quantity and quality of the food that you put on your plate really matters, especially as you look at your dining habits over time.

Follow MyPlate's advice and fill half your plate with fruits and veggies at each meal. Not only will you reduce the total calories that your plate contains, but you will also increase the vitamins, minerals, and fiber you're eating.

In fact, MyPlate is full of good advice. Check out *www.choosemyplate.gov* for details about what foods you should eat and in what quantities. Remember, enjoy your food, but eat less!

Now, before you look at the two plates below, you should know that potatoes are not bad as they appear in the first example. You just need to prepare them in a way that is low in fat and salt. Watching your portion size never hurt either.

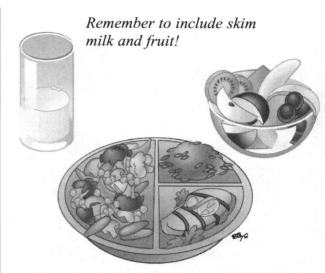

Remember to include skim milk and fruit!

PLATE A - Meat and Potatoes:

Food	Calories	Fat (g)
8 oz fried steak	521	21
6 oz French fries	600	33
Total:	**1121**	**54**

PLATE B - The right mix - 50% vegetables, 25% lean protein, 25% whole grains:

Food	Calories	Fat (g)
1 cup steamed broccoli	54	.55
1 cup steamed carrots	54	.25
4 oz baked chicken breast	140	3.0
1 cup cooked brown rice	108	0.0
Total:	**356**	**4**

Less Fat and More Fiber is Key

A study of U.S. adults age 20-59 years old examined the relationship between diet and Body Mass Index (BMI). The results indicate that, in men, an increased percent of dietary fat was most strongly associated with a greater BMI. While higher fiber was linked with a lower BMI, the association wasn't strong.

By contrast, the women that ate more fiber were much less likely to be overweight or obese. In this case, the link between percent of fat intake and body weight was much weaker than in men, The relative risk that a woman would be overweight or obese is shown in the figure below.[1]

The women who consumed a diet high in fat and fiber were more than three and a half times as likely to be overweight or obese as those who consumed a diet high in fiber and low in fat. However, the women who consumed a lowfat diet that was also low in fiber were about five times as likely to be overweight or obese as those who consumed a low-fat and high-fiber diet.

The data from this study, combined with that collected in other studies, strongly suggests that both men and women would be far less likely to become overweight or obese if they consumed diets with a lot more fiber and a lot less fat than typical diets today.

It should be noted that only about 5% of Americans consume what the newest U.S. Dietary Guidelines called an adequate amount of fiber (14 g per 1,000 calories).

Bottom Line:

A diet made mostly of fruits, vegetables, and whole grains, which is also low in fat and fat-rich foods, helps people lose weight without getting hungry. This is mostly because such a diet has a lower calorie density, less fat, and more fiber, each of which increases feelings of fullness per calorie and thus reduces calorie intake. Such a diet can help people reach adequate intake for fiber, as well as other nutrients. After all, fruits and veggies contain a wide variety of different vitamins and nutrients that can both protect and improve health.

By James J. Kenney, PhD, RD, FACN.

References:

1. *J Am Diet Assoc.* 2005;105:1365-72

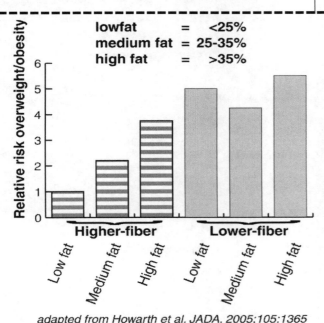

adapted from Howarth et al. JADA. 2005;105:1365

This graph indicates that the risk of becoming overweight/ obese is 4 to 5 times higher when a diet is very low in fiber - even if the fat content of the diet is also fairly low.

This may help to explain why "low-fat" and "fat-free" foods, composed largely of refined flour and sugar, led many to mistakenly believe that high-carbohydrate diets are fattening.

We now know that, in addition to reducing fat in the diet, people also have to cut out most refined carbohydrate-rich foods that are low in fiber, in order to promote weight loss and prevent obesity.

MyPlate: Grains

How many grain foods should I eat?

MyPlate calls for most people to get about 5 to 6 ounce servings of grains per day. At least half of those should be from whole grains. To get a personalized recommendation, visit *www.choosemyplate.gov*.

What is a whole grain?

A whole grain is the entire kernel of a grain, which is made of the bran, endosperm, and germ. Some examples of whole grains include brown rice, popcorn, whole wheat bread, and oatmeal.

What is a refined grain?

Refined grains are made just from the endosperm - the germ and bran are removed. Some examples of refined grains include white flour, white bread, plain pasta, and white rice.

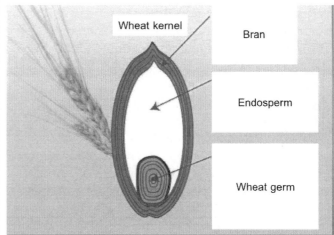

What makes a one ounce serving?

- 1 slice of bread
- 1/2 cup of cooked cereal, rice, or pasta
- 1 ounce of ready-to-eat cereal
- 3 cups of popcorn

		Daily recommendation*	Daily minimum amount of whole grains
Children	2-3 years old	3 ounce equivalents**	1 ½ ounce equivalents**
	4-8 years old	5 ounce equivalents**	2 ½ ounce equivalents**
Girls	9-13 years old	5 ounce equivalents**	3 ounce equivalents**
	14-18 years old	6 ounce equivalents**	3 ounce equivalents**
Boys	9-13 years old	6 ounce equivalents**	3 ounce equivalents**
	14-18 years old	8 ounce equivalents**	4 ounce equivalents**
Women	19-30 years old	6 ounce equivalents**	3 ounce equivalents**
	31-50 years old	6 ounce equivalents**	3 ounce equivalents**
	51+ years old	5 ounce equivalents**	3 ounce equivalents**
Men	19-30 years old	8 ounce equivalents**	4 ounce equivalents**
	31-50 years old	7 ounce equivalents**	3 ½ ounce equivalents**
	51+ years old	6 ounce equivalents**	3 ounce equivalents**

Image from www.choosemyplate.gov/grains-amount.html#

These amounts are for individuals who get less than 30 minutes per day of moderate physical activity. Those who are more physically active may be able to consume more while staying within their daily total calorie needs.

MyPlate: Vegetables

What counts as a vegetable?

- Raw or cooked veggies
- Fresh, frozen, canned, or dried veggies
- Whole, cut-up, or mashed veggies

How many vegetables should I eat each day?

Most people should eat about 2.5 cups per day. To get a personalized recommendation, visit *www.choosemyplate.gov*.

Remember, according to MyPlate, "Eating a diet rich in vegetables and fruits as part of an overall healthy diet may reduce risk for heart disease, including heart attack and stroke."

What counts as a cup?

- 1 cup of raw or cooked vegetables
- 1 cup of 100% vegetable juice
- 2 cups of raw leafy greens

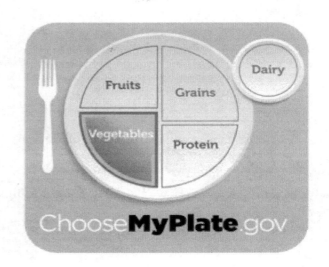

Daily recommendation*		
Children	2-3 years old	1 cup**
	4-8 years old	1½ cups**
Girls	9-13 years old	2 cups**
	14-18 years old	2½ cups**
Boys	9-13 years old	2½ cups**
	14-18 years old	3 cups**
Women	19-30 years old	2½ cups**
	31-50 years old	2½ cups**
	51+ years old	2 cups**
Men	19-30 years old	3 cups**
	31-50 years old	3 cups**
	51+ years old	2½ cups**

This chart is from www.choosemyplate.gov/vegetables-amount.html#

These amounts are for individuals who get less than 30 minutes per day of moderate physical activity. Those who are more physically active may be able to consume more while staying within their daily total calorie needs.

MyPlate: Protein

What is in the protein group?

All foods made from meat, poultry, fish, dry beans or peas, eggs, nuts, and seeds are considered part of this group. Dry beans and peas are also part of the vegetable group. (They're multi-taskers).

Most meat and poultry choices should be lean or low-fat. Fish, nuts, and seeds contain healthy oils, so choose these foods more often than meat or poultry. According to MyPlate, "Seafood contains a range of nutrients, notably the omega-3 fatty acids, EPA and DHA." Eat a wide variety of protein foods.

Proteins help build your muscles, skin, cartilage, bones, and even blood. They also aid the development of enzymes and hormones.

How much is needed each day?

Most Americans eat enough food from this group, but need to make leaner and more varied shoices.

Recommended daily amounts are shown in the chart below. Most people should eat about 5 to 6 ounces per day. Try to get a few small servings of different kinds of protein every day. For a personalized recommendation, visit *www.choosemyplate.gov*.

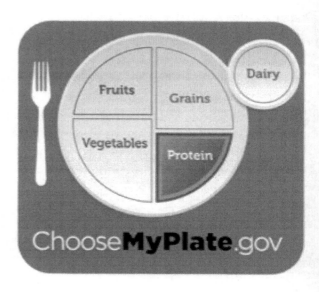

What counts as an ounce?

- 1 ounce of meat, poultry or fish
- 1/4 cup of cooked dry beans
- 1 egg
- 1 tablespoon of peanut butter
- 1/2 ounce of nuts or seeds

Daily recommendation*		
Children	2-3 years old	2 ounce equivalents**
	4-8 years old	4 ounce equivalents**
Girls	9-13 years old	5 ounce equivalents**
	14-18 years old	5 ounce equivalents**
Boys	9-13 years old	5 ounce equivalents**
	14-18 years old	6 ½ ounce equivalents**
Women	19-30 years old	5 ½ ounce equivalents**
	31-50 years old	5 ounce equivalents**
	51+ years old	5 ounce equivalents**
Men	19-30 years old	6 ½ ounce equivalents**
	31-50 years old	6 ounce equivalents**
	51+ years old	5 ½ ounce equivalents**

Image from www.choosemyplate.gov/protein-foods-amount.html#

These amounts are for individuals who get less than 30 minutes per day of moderate physical activity. Those who are more physically active may be able to consume more while staying within their daily total calorie needs.

Making the Best Choices

Many people stick to the same old meat or poultry choices in order to get the protein they need every day. It is important to vary foods in this group so that you eat fish, beans, nuts, and seeds on a more regular basis.

Include fish, nuts, and seeds for essential fats and better heart health. A wide variety of protein foods will also help you get vital nutrients.

Meat and Poultry

Start with a lean choice:

- The leanest beef cuts include round steaks and roasts (round eye, top round, bottom round, round tip), top loin, top sirloin, and chuck shoulder and arm roasts.

- The leanest pork choices include pork loin, tenderloin, center loin, and ham.

- Choose extra lean ground beef or ground turkey breast without skin. It helps to rinse ground meat after cooking to remove excess grease.

- The leanest choice for chicken or turkey is breast meat without the skin.

Keep it lean:

- Trim all visible fat before cooking.

- Prepare items with little fat. Broil, grill, roast, or poach meat, poultry, or fish instead of frying.

- Drain off any fat that appears during cooking.

- Skip or limit the breading on meat, poultry, or fish. Breading adds fat and calories. It will also cause the food to soak up more fat during the frying process.

- Use sauces or gravies that are low in fat. Consider using a de-fatter cup on homemade gravy.

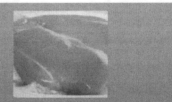

Keep It Low in Fat

Choose lean cuts of meat

Select white poultry without skin

Use low-fat preparation methods

Fish

Choose fish more often for lunch or dinner. Look for fish rich in omega-3 fatty acids, such as salmon, trout, and herring. Try...

- Salmon steaks or filets
- Canned salmon in water
- Grilled or baked trout

Beans and Peas

Make beans and peas a central part of several meals per week. Want some ideas? Try...

- Chili with kidney or pinto beans
- A stir fry dish with tofu
- Bean soups
- Baked beans
- Garbanzo beans on a salad
- Rice and beans
- Veggie burgers
- Hummus spread on pita bread

Nuts and Seeds

Choose nuts as a snack, on salads, or in main dishes. Use nuts to replace meat or poultry, not in addition to these items. Be sure to eat them in small quantities. After all, they do still have a lot of fat.

Quiz: Build a Healthier Plate

1. Pick the most heart-healthy protein choice:
a. Medium cheeseburger
b. Fried chicken breast
c. 3 ounces of baked salmon
d. They are all good choices

2. Which protein is the highest in fiber and lowest in calories?
a. Black beans
b. Pork tenderloin, gravy
c. Pan-fried trout
d. Fried fish sandwich

3. You should fill your plate about half full with a lean animal protein item, leaving the rest of the space for a starch.
a. True
b. False

4. If you had the following breakfast choices, which would be the best one?
a. Vegetable omelette
b. Biscuit and gravy
c. Oatmeal with skim milk
d. Bagel with cream cheese

5. Which grain is the best choice for your heart?
a. Whole-wheat pasta
b. Brown rice
c. Barley
d. They are all good choices

6. About three fourths of your plate should be filled with fruits, vegetables and whole grains.
a. True
b. False

7. Which vegetables are best for your heart?
a. Broccoli
b. Carrots
c. They are both good choices

8. Three ounces of meat/fish or chicken is about the size of a:
a. Deck of cards
b. Golf ball
c. Man's shoe

9. You are given a choice of the following side dishes... which one is lowest in fat?
a. Baked potato
b. French fries
c. Onion rings

10. How many vegetables should most people eat each day?
a. One cup
b. Two cups
c. Half a cup

Answers:
1. C (salmon) 2. A (black beans)
3. B (false) 4. C (oatmeal, skim milk)
5. D (they are all good choices)
6. A (true) 7. C (they are all good choices) 8. A (deck of cards)
9. A (baked potato or sweet potato)
10. B (2 cups)

Score:
Tally up your score. How did you do?
• 8-10 answers right: A - You are right on!
• 6-8 answers right: B - You need a little work.
• 4-5 answers right: C - You need more work.
• 1-3 answers right: D - Uh oh, try again.
For more information about healthful eating and activities, visit *ChooseMyPlate.gov*.

Work Out When You Are Stressed

Overeating is just one of the ways that we cope with daily pressures. The next time you find yourself reaching for a snack, consider exercising instead.

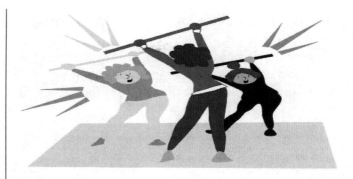

Exercise - The Natural Stress Reducer

When you experience stress, your body releases certain chemicals. Exercise burns off these chemicals and allows your body to relax. It also improves sleep and boosts your immune system. Did you know that lack of exercise actually stresses your body? Without exercise, your flexibility, overall strength, and muscle tone will all decrease.

Regular Exercise Improves Your Mood

Exercise burns calories and makes you feel better. It improves concentration and produces endorphins, the body' natural pain reliever. Studies have even proven that exercise can relieve depression.

Exercise Doesn't Have To Be Hard

Exercise at school can include walking, climbing stairs, or just stretching between classes. At home, exercise can consist of gardening, mowing the lawn, practicing sports, riding your bike to a friend's house, etc. Try walking an extra lap at the mall before you shop. Ride your bike to a nearby grocery store. Find something you enjoy and stick with it!

Replace "Happy Hour" with an "Exercise Hour"

If going out for a snack after school is how and your friends unwind after a stressful day, consider an alternative. Instead of adding extra calories to your day, plan to exercise instead. Meet your friends for a walk, a bike ride, or a trip to the local health club. You'll feel relaxed and happy that you didn't overindulge.

Get Away From the Food Source

Your workout can take you away from the kitchen, pre-meal snacking, or whatever eating cues you find difficult to resist. Exercising between school and your evening meal gives you even more benefits. You'll save "snacking" calories before dinner, burn some of the calories that you already consumed, and may even eat less for dinner. Sometimes exercise can reduce your appetite.

Eat Because You Are Hungry

Exercise burns calories, which your body will want to restore. That means that when you eat, you'll be eating for a reason, not just because it's time to eat. Regular exercisers have been shown to eat healthier than those who don't exercise. After working hard to burn calories, it's more difficult to reach for food that doesn't meet your nutritional needs.

Working Out - A Great Alternative to "Doing Nothing"

Don't let boredom be your reason for overeating. Replace your afternoon snack with an aerobic routine. Exercise gives you something constructive to do with your free time. Consider saving up for a piece of home exercise equipment. Then, this winter, you can watch your favorite TV show while you exercise. As you become more fit, exercise may even become something you want to do. Make it a habit.

What Are Your Sources of Stress?

Stress Quiz - What Are Your Sources of Stress?

Stress is our body's reaction to everyday experiences and unexpected changes. Review these stress sources and check off the ones that apply to you.

Change in school assignments   _____

Death of a family   _____

Debt (your family's or your own)   _____

Depression/mental health issues   _____

Parents' divorce or separation   _____

Family problems   _____

General health concerns   _____

Upcoming weddings   _____

Holidays   _____

Legal concerns   _____

New sibling   _____

New house   _____

New school   _____

Time (not enough)   _____

School (in general)   _____

School and life balance   _____

Stress Symptoms - Which Ones Are You Feeling?

Stress is a normal part of life. It can be good or bad. Both a wedding and a funeral will cause our body to react in the same way (in terms of chemicals and stress hormones). Constant stress leads to anxiety and unhealthy behaviors like overeating.

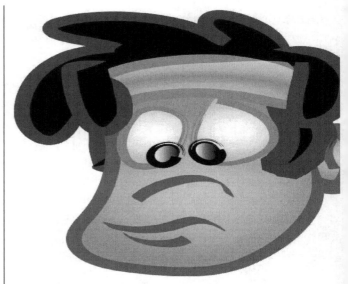

Stress Symptoms

These are some of the symptoms you may experience if you have high levels of stress:

- Recurring headaches, stomach problems, or backaches
- Short fuse – either anger or tears more often than usual
- Impatience or frustration in normal situations
- Feelings of loneliness
- Frequent illnesses, injuries, or accidents
- Failure to concentrate
- Excessive fatigue or lack of focus
- Muscular tension
- Anxiety (sweating, dry mouth, twitching, etc)
- Dizziness
- Irritability
- Digestive problems
- Sadness or depression (seek help in this circumstance)

Building Resiliance to Manage Stress

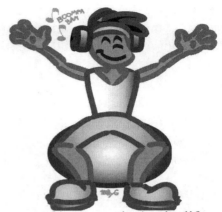

Resilience is a measure of how quickly you can bounce back when things go wrong in your life. A wide variety of things affect how you react under stress, but it is possible to increase your resilience by adjusting the ways you choose to cope, as well as how you view the situation. Think of it this way – resiliance is part of who you are, while stress management is part of what you do. Here are some tips to help you improve your resilience and resist the temptation to overeat:

- Resilient people have **self-confidence**: Learning to believe in yourself will provide you with a buffer against people who say or do hurtful things. Building your self-confidence can include trying new challenges and, eventually, succeeding at them. Get involved in clubs, crafts, church, or other activities. Find a place where you can voice your opinion or do something with others. Surround yourself with people who like you for who you are.

- Resilient people are **optimistic**: Optimistic people have better health, live longer, and have more success in life. Expect the best instead of the worst. Thinking positive makes it easier to deal with life's unexpected bumps.

- Resilient people have **friends** and good relationships: Friends and family allow you to express your feelings. Standing up for yourself with those you love makes it easier to do the same in the "real world." Don't let anyone take advantage of you, but get involved when you can help. Doing things for your friends and family will make you feel like you belong to a community.

- Resilient people **enjoy life**: Take time each day to do something your enjoy. It may include art, sports, crafts, or other activities. Be open to learning new things. Find something good in life's difficulties. Have a good time wherever you go. You should also main-

tain a sense of humor – don't take life so seriously. Adjust to change instead of dreading it. Learn to do things in a new and different way.

- Resilient people trust their **intuition**: Go with your gut. It may not always lead you perfectly, but it generally has a good track record. Relying on your instincts will help build your self- confidence.

- Resilient people have **perseverance**: If at first you don't succeed, don't give up. Believe in your ability to succeed. Resilient people set goals and take the steps to achieve them. To become more resilient, practice finishing the tasks that you set out to do

- Resilient people have **good life skills**: Set a goal and take steps to achieve it. Pursue extra training to prepare you for college and your adult life. Use honest and open communication to solve the problems in your life. When conflicts arise, solve them in ways that don't compromise your values.

- Resilient people **take care of themselves**: Maintain your health with good nutrition. This should include fruits and vegetables, lean meats or fish, whole grains, and lowfat dairy products. Limit your consumption of caffeine. Exercise and lift weights regularly to maintain your overall strength. Practice relaxation methods. Limit your exposure to stressful situations. Be good to your body.

Avoid Hidden Calories

- Keep a calorie diary for a week. Look at the times that you consume hidden calories, then change your routine to avoid falling into the habit.
- Count the hidden calories that you are eating. You'll find it harder to ignore these calories once you know how many you are consuming.
- Practice portion control when you are eating snacks. Put together your own 100-calorie packs, then limit yourself to one bag when you decide to snack.
- Eat before a big party or celebration. If you are bringing food, be sure to bring something that you like that won't blow your calorie budget.
- Get more exercise on the days that you overeat. You may not burn off all of the calories you consumed, but it will help!
- Find something else to do in place of eating. Keep away from situations that cause you to overeat.
- Drink something low calorie or chew gum when you aren't busy.

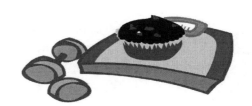

Home	What	Might Include
Cooking calories	Sampling food	Eating entrees, cookie dough
After school calories	Snacking while unaware	Cookies, candies, chips
Celebration calories	Cooking high calorie foods	Tasting foods high in calories
On the run caloires	Eating in the car	Fast food
Candy calories	Fundraiser items	Candy in the house
Phone calories	Eating snacks	Eating a lot when distracted
Parties		
Food table calories	Hanging out by the food table	Being unaware of the calories you ate
Snack calories	Snack bowls everywhere	Grabbing snacks as you pass
Drink calories	Want to belong	Choosing high calorie drinks
Restaurant		
Bread calories	Hard to quit eating	Eating until bread basket is gone
Drink calories	Want to drink something	Ordering beverages with calories
Dessert calories	Want to indulge	Very high calorie end to meal

Do You Have Cues to Overeat?

What are *Your* Cues To Overeat?

People overeat for a variety of reasons. Many overeat because of stress, not because they are actually hungry. Here is a list of some of the cues to overeat, along with ways to cope with those cues:

Recreational Eating:

Birthdays, holidays, parties, school events, or other special occasions are times when overeating is encouraged and expected – the temptations are everywhere and the stakes are high. After all, your friends and family want you to join in the fun. When you find yourself with people that you don't know, it's sometimes easier to overeat than to talk with them. In order to limit overeating:

Keep away from the food as much as possible.

- Make healthy choices when you are away from home. Try to limit your portion sizes. When possible, bring your own food.
- Avoid being near foods that you normally binge on. Don't take second helpings from the buffet table. Arrive late or leave early to limit your contact time with food. Help out with setup or decorations instead of overeating.

"Bad Times" Eating:

When we experience stressful situations, we tend to use food as a way to cope. Since something major in our lives is different, we tend to feel uncomfortable, especially at first.

- Take care of yourself to make overeating less likely. Get some extra exercise. Plan to do something special for yourself during stressful periods. Get a massage, some new exercise clothes, game tickets, or a new haircut.
- Some people eat when they feel bad about themselves. Whether someone says something bad about you, you make a mistake at school, or you confront a friend about a difference of opinion, you may leave the situation feeling unhappy with yourself. Afterward, you could end up binge eating to cope. Instead of blaming yourself for everything, try to put it in perspective. Will what bothered you today bother you in a month? Are you blowing what happened out of proportion?
- Call a friend or someone you can talk to before you overeat. Changing your attitude about yourself will help you avoid overeating in the future.

Irregular Eating:

Skipping meals, making poor nutritional choices, and eating on the run can cause you to overeat.

- Eating regular meals can help you avoid overeating. Keep your food in the portions and proportions that MyPlate outlines.
- Make sure to eat a variety of foods from all the food groups. This will keep you healthy and help you cope with stress. For a personalized recommendation about what you should eat each day, visit *www.choosemyplate.gov*.

Missing Foods You Love:

Most weight loss plans remove many of the foods that you enjoy eating. When your willpower is low, you may return to the foods you love, but eat too many of them. After all, you haven't had them for a long time. Your weight loss plan should include the foods you love in small doses and on occasion. As a result, you will not feel deprived and you'll be less likely to binge eat.

Boredom:

Many people eat when they want something to do. Watching TV or surfing the web often go hand in hand with snacking. When you do two activities at once, you tend to eat larger quantities of food, especially when you aren't paying particular attention to portion size.

Find something else to do in place of eating. Consider working on a craft while watching TV. Go for a walk during commercial breaks instead of snacking.

Ways to Avoid Overeating

Avoid Overeating

There are many ways to cope with stress instead of overeating. Here are a few ideas:

Do Something for Yourself:

- Learn how to do progressive deep relaxation. Do this instead of overeating.
- Listen to music.
- Take a long bath.
- Get a massage
- Go out with some friends.
- Buy yourself some flowers.
- Get a haircut.
- Take a new exercise class.

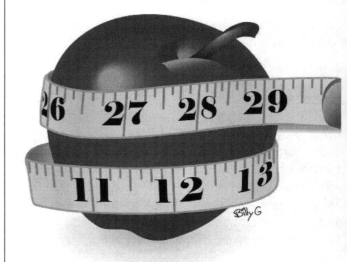

Find Good Alternatives to Overeating

- Purchase books or magazines. Go somewhere pleasant to read them and avoid eating.
- Join a health club. Make a commitment to exercise 3-5 times each week. Find a partner to exercise with and keep you motivated.
- Take a class and learn a new craft. This will keep your hands busy while you watch TV, surf the web, or talk on the phone.
- Leave the house to avoid excess eating.
- Take a couple of laps around the mall before or after dinner.
- Mow the lawn.
- Weed the garden.
- Clean your room.
- Consider saving up for a piece of home exercise equipment. Exercise while you watch TV.
- Lift weights while you watch TV

Manage Your Stress

- Be aware of your stressors.
- Reduce your emotional reaction to stress. Take a deep breath and try to relax.
- Practice how to deal with major stressors in your life.
- Learn what you can change. Decide what is worth fighting for.
- Build up your physical reserves. Take care of yourself by:
  - Cutting back on caffeine during times of stress.
  - Eating healthy meals. Be sure you are meeting your nutritional needs. Visit www.*choosemyplate.gov* if you aren't sure about what you should be eating.
  - Get enough sleep. If you have difficulty sleeping, see a professional.
  - Have some fun. Take vacations and leave your stresses at home.
  - Learn to say no. It's ok to take care of your own needs.
  - Include friends and family in your life, regardless of how busy you are.
  - Set realistic goals for yourself.
  - Expect some bumps in the road. Things will get better over time.

Should Cravings Be Your Guide?

Guys and girls crave different foods

Chocolate is the most often reported craving for women. Men are more likely to report cravings for meats and salty snack foods. Since nearly all the foods craved by guys and girls are calorie dense, it is not surprising to find overweight people reporting intense food cravings.

Eating too few calories may backfire

Since eating too little or seriously reducing the calories you eat increases hunger, and hunger increases the desire to eat all foods, it is not surprising that people on super low calorie diets often end up overdoing it on a preferred food.

Cravings reflect a desire for pleasure

Many people believe that a craving or desire for a specific food is an indication of nutritional need. Some researchers have suggested that, since most cravings are for nutrient poor foods that are high in fat, sugar and/or salt, such cravings are unlikely to have anything to do with real nutritional needs. These researchers note that food items that are delicious are the most likely to be craved. The researchers believe that most food cravings simply reflect a desire for comfort; often people who are depressed, anxious, or lonely report the most intense food cravings.

The more fat you eat, the more you crave

Other researchers note that certain neurotransmitters increase the desire to eat certain types of food. For example, galanin increases the desire for fatty foods, while neuropeptide Y is associated with a desire for high carbohydrate foods. Research also indicates that, the more fat in one's diet, the more galanin is produced. The more galanin that's produced, the more one prefers or craves fattier foods. Indeed, research shows that eating less fat for several weeks reduces galanin levels and the desire to eat fatty foods.

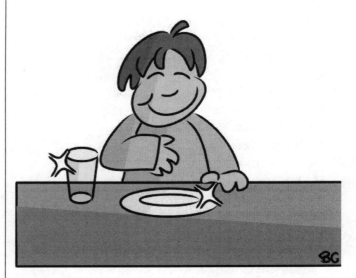

Avoid the foods you crave in order to eat less of them

It is clear that the only way to reduce a desire for fatty foods is to not eat said foods. There is no evidence that avoiding a certain food will create a more intense craving or desire to eat that food. In fact, avoidance is the only proven way to reduce one's desire for a craved food item.

Contrary to popular myth, food cravings do not reflect a real nutritional need and often undermine rational attempts to improve one's diet. In general, the only way to reduce the desire for unhealthy foods is to avoid them for several weeks. With time, such cravings get smaller and become easier to control.

By Dr. James J. Kenney, PhD, RD, FACN
Reprinted from Communicating Food for Health
Newsletter.

50 Things to Do When Bored Besides Eat

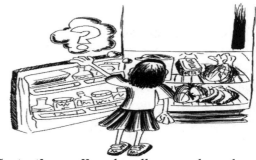

1. **Plan healthy meals and snacks**. Keep a healthful routine and do not choose calorie-dense foods at random.
2. Ask your parents to help you **stock the house with good, healthy foods**.
3. Clean out the **refrigerator** and freezer.
4. **Drink water** or unsweetened tea.
5. **Clean the house** or catch up on chores.
6. **Wash the car**.
7. **Clean the back yard** or patio, if you have one.
8. Go to the **gym**.
9. If you find you have a lot of extra time on your hands, enroll in an **exercise class**.
10. **Organize your closet** and donate extra items to charity.
11. **Prepare a low-fat salad** and raw vegetable snacks for the day or week.
12. **Walk the dog** (or a neighbor's dog, if you don't have one).
13. **Get ready the night before** so that you will have time to exercise the next morning.
14. **Go out for unsweetened tea or coffee**.
15. **Shop for gifts** and get ahead with your life schedule so that you have more time for exercise.
16. **Learn a new, healthful recipe** that features fruit or vegetables.
17. **Prepare a healthy dinner**.
18. **Cut up fruit and put grapes in small baggies** so that they are ready to go.
19. **Take up swimming**, biking, hiking, kayaking, or another physical activity.
20. Buy and use an **exercise video**.
21. Find a **yoga studio** and take two lessons a week.
22. **Call a friend** and walk around while you are talking on the phone.
23. **Chew gum** or brush your teeth.
24. **Write down** situations that cause you stress and make you want to eat, then find non-food alternative activities.
25. **Reorganize your bathroom** or other areas in the house.
26. **Drink water** flavored with lemon.
27. **Talk a long walk** to the store.
28. **Go to the mall** and walk around, or do outdoor shopping.
29. **Walk around the zoo** or outdoor park.
30. **Shop online** for new fitness equipment and clothes.
31. Write down what you have eaten today and **start a food journal**.
32. **Make a list of the times you feel bored** and need to eat, then make a list of things that you can do to conquer this feeling.
33. **Research and write inspirational quotes**.
34. **Listen to music** while taking a walk.
35. **Organize your photographs**.
36. **Catch up on your email**.
37. **Meditate** or take a hot bath, and then pamper yourself by making sure that you look good.
38. **Ride an exercise bike while you watch TV**. It is even better if you can watch a show or DVD that features an inspirational athletic event.
39. **Sign up for tennis lessons**.
40. Go **bowling**.
41. **Volunteer** so that you are out of the house and around people more often.
42. **Cook some healthful low-fat meals** and freeze them for busy days.
43. **Organize your kitchen**.
44. **Attend an outdoor farmer's market**.
45. Go out **dancing**.
46. Write down **goals** for yourself for the coming year - budget, vacation, school, lifestyle, etc.
47. Eat **carrots**, celery, or melon.
48. **Iron** your clothes.
49. Go to the **bookstore**.
50. Take some outdoor **photographs**.

Chocolate Craving Solutions

Here are some lower-calorie ideas and tips for chocolate cravings.

- Cocoa powder is a low fat substitute for chocolate. Sprinkle it over lowfat frozen yogurt (remember to measure the yogurt, 1 portion = 1/2 cup).
- For the least fat, try York Peppermint Patties, Junior Mints, Kit Kat Bars, Hershey's Sweet Escapes, or 3 Musketeers to satisfy your chocolate craving (remember to read serving size info).
- Fit your "budgeted" chocolate serving into a balanced, heart-healthy, high fiber, low fat diet.
- Eat dark chocolate to satisfy your craving in fewer bites.
- Select a small chocolate biscotti from your favorite coffee house.
- Avoid large portions of dessert, cookies, and brownies. Avoid large chocolate bars. These all contain upwards of 400 calories, with some totalling as many as 1000 calories per serving!

Banana Sundae

1 large banana

1 tablespoon fat-free whipped cream

1 tablespoon light chocolate syrup

1 teaspoon sprinkles

Peel banana and cut in half lengthwise, then place in a dessert dish or bowl.

Top banana with chocolate syrup and a little whipped cream. Lightly coat the top of the whipped cream with sprinkles. Serve immediately.

Servings:

Serves 1. Each serving: 1 banana: 155 calories, 1 g fat, 0 g saturated fat, 0 g trans fat, 2 mg cholesterol, 24 mg sodium, 38 g carbohydrate, 3 g fiber, 2 g protein.

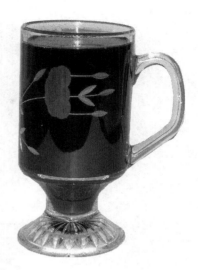

Light Chocolate Mousse

12 ounces silken tofu

1/3 cup Splenda

1/4 cup cocoa powder

1/3 cup skim milk

2 tablespoons whipped cream

Blend tofu, Splenda, and cocoa powder in a food processor until smooth. Place chocolate mousse in four individual serving dishes (about 2/3 cup per serving). Chill before serving.

Optional: Top with whipped cream when ready to serve.

Servings: Makes 4 - 1 cup servings. Each serving: 99 calories, 4.5 g fat, 0 g saturated fat, 0 g trans fat, 2 mg cholesterol, 41 mg sodium, 8 g carbohydrate, 0 g fiber, 7 g protein.

Fresh berries with chocolate sauce

1/2 cup fresh berries

1 tablespoon chocolate syrup

Drizzle the berries with chocolate syrup.

Serves 1. Each 1/2 cup serving: 114 calories, 1 g fat, 0 g saturated fat, 0 g trans fat, 2 mg cholesterol, 24 mg sodium, 28 g carbohydrate, 3 g fiber, 1 g protein.

Made in the USA
Middletown, DE
12 November 2015